COMPANION BOOK TO THE GUIDING STAR CYCLE SHOW

WHAT'S GOING ON IN MY BODY?

All About the Female Cycle, Periods, and Fertility

Elisabeth Raith-Paula, MD

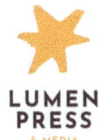

LUMEN
PRESS
& MEDIA

WHAT'S GOING ON IN MY BODY?
All About the Female Cycle, Periods, and Fertility
By Elisabeth Raith-Paula, MD

Copyright ©2023 Lumen Press. All rights reserved. It is not permitted to scan, save on PCs or any other computers, change or manipulate any illustrations of this book, unless with written permission of Elisabeth Raith-Paula and Lumen Press. Except for brief quotations for review purposes, no part of this book may be reproduced in any form without prior written permission from the author.

Original Copyright © Elisabeth Raith-Paula ISBN 978-3-00-058549-4
The original German version: "Was ist los in meinem Körper?" and the Copyright
© 2019 Knaur Verlag An imprint of Verlagsgruppe Droemer Knaur GmbH & Ko.KG, München

Photo Credits
Cover Photo: @Jupiterimages from Photo Images via Canva.com
Photos: iStock by Getty Images p. 9, p. 10 / Raith-Paula p. 11 top / iStock by Getty Images p.11 bottom / iStock by Getty Images p. 13 / Raith-Paula p. 15/ iStock by Getty Images p.17 , p.19, p. 24, p. 26 top and bottom, p. 29 top and bottom / Raith-Paula p. 30, p. 34, p 35 / iStock by Getty Images p. 37 middle and bottom / Raith-Paula p. 39 / iStock by Getty Images p. 40 / Raith-Paula p. 42 / iStock by Getty Images p. 43 , p. 46, p. 49 / Raith-Paula p. 50 / iStock by Getty Images p. 53, p. 54 / Raith-Paula p. 57 / iStock by Getty Images p. 58, p. 59, p. 60, p. 63, p. 66, p. 69, p. 70, p. 74 / Anna Flynn p. 75 / iStock by Getty Images p. 78, p. 83 / Raith-Paula p. 87 / iStock by Getty Images p. 89, p. 91, p. 100, p. 101, p. 106, p. 108 / Raith-Paula p. 111 / iStock by Getty Images p. 114, p. 117 , p. 129.

Original Composition and Layout Design: Zsolt Halasi
2023 Updates to Composition and Layout Edits: Sarah Ward
American Cover Layout Design: Sarah Ward (The Art Ward) • ArtWardStudio@gmail.com
Translation: Geraldine Groll and Hilary Hodgson
Editing: Sarah Hughes
American English Editing: Elessa Marker
Illustrations: "Ente" Andreas Endres (rights for illustrations: Elisabeth Raith-Paula)

To contact the publisher: contact@theguidingstarproject.com
To purchase copies visit: www.LumenPress.org
To contact the author: Elisabeth Raith-Paula • www.mfm-projekt.eu • info@mfm-projekt.de

ISBN (Print): 978-1-7352237-6-6

Dedication

This book is dedicated to my daughter Marion and all girls whom I'm allowed to accompany during the exciting years in which they develop from a girl to a woman.

Acknowledgement

Thank you Hilary—only because of your tireless commitment and hard work this book now becomes a reality. Thanks also to Jenny for your proofreading and your helpful suggestions and kind support on chapter two and ten.

Table of Contents

Introduction: A Handbook for Becoming a Woman — 7

1 Secret Signs — 8
The "Three Corners Game" – Tricky Questions — 8
Are You Fertile Today? — 9
What Do You Think of When You Hear the Word "Fertility?" — 10

2 The Equation of Life – Sperm + Egg = Baby — 12
The Sperm – 1,000 per Second! — 12
The Egg – Rare and Precious — 15
Preparations for a Special Guest — 16
On the Stage of Life — 17

3 The Equation of Life – How a New Life Begins — 21
The Adventurous Journey of the Sperm — 21
"And the winner is…." – Fertilization — 26
It's all about Timing – Fertile or Not Fertile? — 31

4 Clear the Stage for the Cycle Show — 33
The Control Center – The Brain Regulates Hormones — 33
First Act of the Cycle Show – Estrogens Start Working — 34
Second Act of the Cycle Show – The Service Center Goes into Action — 38
Grand Finale and Small Finale — 42

5 Puberty and the Premiere of the Cycle Show — 46
The Cycle Show Section is Open – Puberty Begins — 46
Estrogens Transform a Girl into a Woman — 47
Changes on the Stage of Life — 50
The Premiere: The First Period, the Menarche — 52

6 The Small Finale – My Period — 58
Blood is the Essence of Life — 59
What's Really Happening in the Body — 61
Different than Usual — 63
Make the Days of Your Period Special — 66
Period Products– It's Up to You — 68

7 Looking for my Body's Secret Code — 71
Observing the Physical Signs — 71
Body Code: Cervical Mucus – "Discharge" or a "Magic Potion" — 73
Body Code: Temperature Shift – The Progesterone Team Turn

    Up the Heat   78
Body Code: Cervix –
    The Gate of Life   82
Body Code: Ovulation Pain –
    Happiness can Sometimes Hurt   85
Body Code: Ovulation Bleeding –
    A Little Blood at the Time
    of Ovulation   86
Body Code: Breast Symptoms –
    The Overeager Progesterone Team   87
More Body Codes –
    Entirely Individual   88

8 Cycle Length and Cycle Variation – When Am I Fertile?   91

What Exactly Do We Mean
    by Regular?   91
First Act Varies, the Second
    is Constant   94
When Am I Fertile?   95

9 The Cycle Show Put to the Test – Various Types of Cycles and Their Causes   100

Stress Type A: Delayed Ripening
    of the Egg   102
Stress Type B: Cycle without Ovulation   103
Stress Type C: Shortened Luteal Phase   105
Stress type D: No More Periods   106

10 The Effect of Different Contraceptive Methods on a Woman's Body   109

The Equation of Life is No Longer Valid   110
Combined Oral Contraception (COC/Birth
    Control Pill) –
    The Effect on the Cycle Show   110
Progestogen Only Contraceptive
    Methods   121
The Copper Intrauterine Device (Cu-IUD)
    –
    The Copper Coil   126
The Emergency Pill   128

11 It's All a Matter of Timing   131

Appendix – Information about the MFM Project   135

Information about the Guiding Star Cycle Show Workshop   136

Important Terms and Definitions   139

Index   142

Additional Resources   144

A Handbook for Becoming a Woman

The aim of this book is to accompany you during the exciting years in which you develop from a girl into a woman.

In chapters one to seven, you will begin by finding out about the changes in your body. What is it like to have your first period and what is your body telling you when this occurs? You will come to understand that the changes you notice are important signs of what is happening inside of you, enabling you to get to know your body and yourself better.

It's quite possible that your body seems a little alien to you at the moment. You may have already noticed some changes and are not quite sure what to make of it or whether you want it to change at all. This book will help you to decipher your body's secret signs, empowering you with knowledge so that you can feel proud to become a woman.

There may be times when you're not feeling so great and are perhaps worried that something is going wrong with your body or your menstrual cycle. Chapters eight and nine of this book will help you during these times by explaining the amazing things that are taking place inside of your body.

At a later stage of your life, you will undoubtedly have questions about fertility and contraception and want to gather lots of information from friends, the internet, brochures and health professionals. This would also be the perfect opportunity to take this book out again and read the final section. Chapters ten and eleven explain a woman's fertile time and when she can become pregnant in more detail, as well as the effect that various methods of hormonal contraception have on a woman's body. Knowing how it is possible to live in harmony with your body will enable you to make decisions that are best for you.

After all, you'll know exactly what's going on in your body!

Take a Deeper Dive into the Book

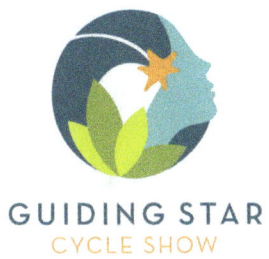

Are you looking for more resources in order to dive deeper into the wonders of the developing female body? Look no further!

The Guiding Star Cycle Show team have created a variety of interactive and fun activity pages to further engage you, your daughter, and/or the students you work with as they discover the wonders of their female bodies. And better yet, ALL of these resources are FREE to you with the purchase of this book. Scan the QR code below to access these downloadable resources to work through with the young girls in your life or allow them to dive deeper on their own time.

New resources will be continued to be developed and added for downloadable access so be sure to subscribe to our email list so you know when the next resource is available to you.

1 Secret Signs

The "Three Corners Game" – Tricky Questions

Try to imagine you're standing in an empty room. In the room there is a "yes," a "no," and an "I don't know" corner. Someone asks you a question, and instead of giving a response, you have to go to a corner of the room. Ok, let´s get started!

The first question is: "Are you hungry?"
"What a silly question", you think to yourself. "I've just had a big breakfast, so no, I'm not hungry", and you go and stand in the "no" corner. How would you know if you're hungry? That's easy! Your tummy would rumble and the empty feeling in your stomach would have you heading straight for the fridge.

Next question: "Are you thirsty?"
"Yes I am", you think, and head over to the "yes" corner. Where did you learn to recognize a feeling of thirst? Did you learn it as a baby or at school? The truth is, it's not really something one needs to learn, your mouth simply feels dry and your tongue seems to stick to the roof of your mouth. Thirst is pretty obvious, even babies realize it.

Onto the next question: "Do you have a favorite pop star?" You think to yourself, "Yes I do!" so you go to the "Yes" corner. What would happen if the door opened this very minute and your favorite pop star came in and walked straight up to you? How would you feel about that? The very thought of it could give you goose bumps, butterflies in your stomach, sweaty hands, make your knees shake, and your heart thump. Unfortunately, it's not possible to fulfill that dream right now, but do you notice how your body reacts just at the very thought of it? The body's messages are very clear: hunger, thirst, excitement and nervousness.

Wait, you're not quite finished yet! Back to the reality of everyday life and the next question: "Do you need to go to the bathroom?"

You do need to go, so you head straight to the "yes" corner. But hang on a minute, how do you know that? Yet another silly

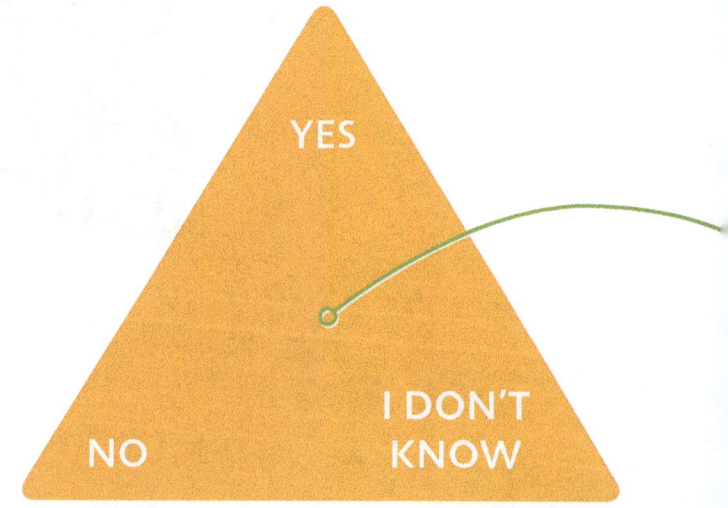

question! It's obvious isn't it? It's that feeling of pressure from your bladder, which suddenly we're all able to locate exactly within our body without any medical knowledge. Why? For the simple reason that it is the bladder that sends out a signal that makes it clear to everyone: "Now I need to go to the bathroom.

Are You Fertile Today?

The final question: "Are you fertile today, at this very moment?"

Your response might be something like "Huh? What's that supposed to mean?! How should I know? What does "fertile" mean anyway? Whether I could get pregnant? Have children? That's a strange question, is it even possible to know the answer?"

You go to the "I don't know" corner for the first time. Up until now all the other questions were so easy to answer, however the body does send clear signals to say "today I'm fertile" or "today I'm not fertile" just like it does with hunger and thirst.

A woman's body goes through a number of changes, over and over again each month. The changes we see on the outside give us important information about the changes that are happening inside, acting like signals or messages to tell you a great deal about yourself. If you know how

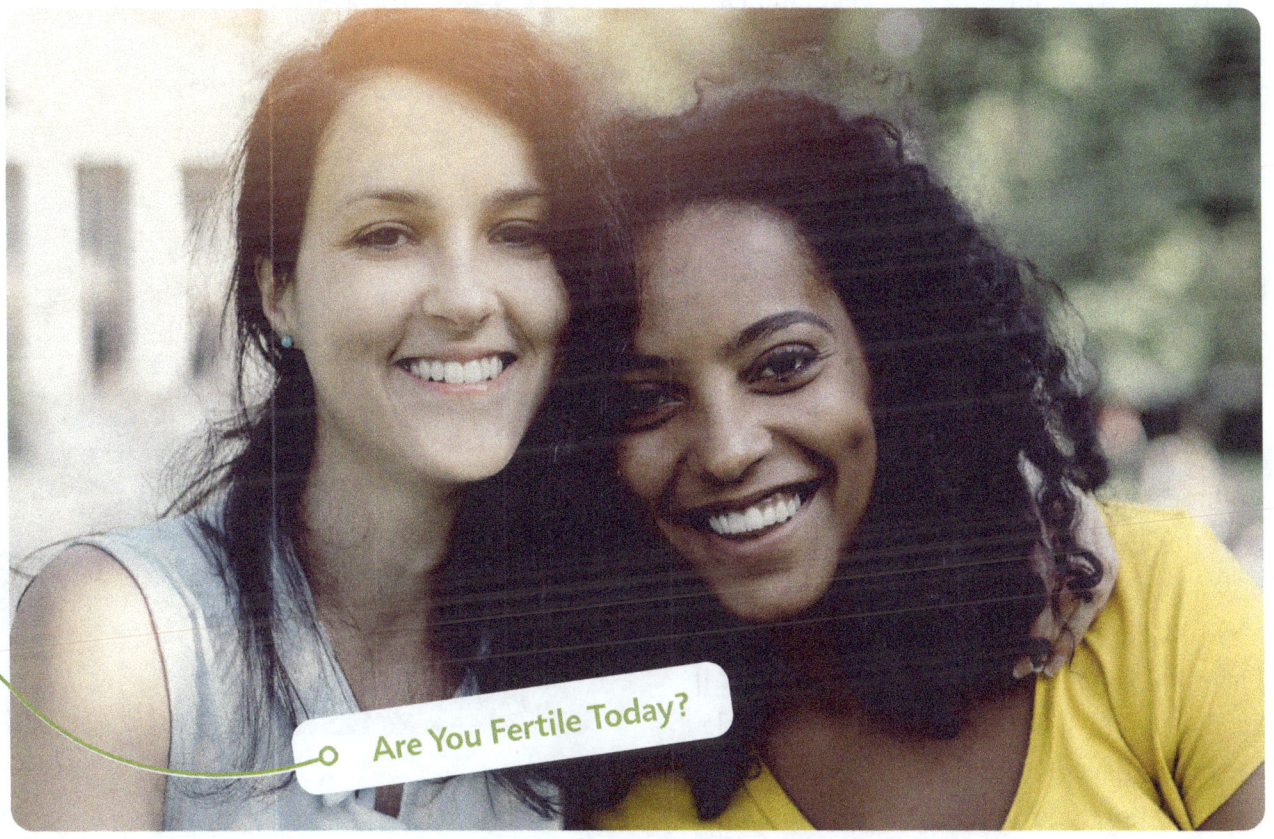

Are You Fertile Today?

to understand the signals correctly, then it allows you to recognize what is going on in your body at that moment, and can even help you understand your feelings, moods and emotions.

The strange thing is that these signals often go unnoticed. Even when we detect that something is happening, we seldom know what it means. This is why we often completely misunderstand our body's signals, when actually all it's telling us is that everything is just fine.

It's time we start to correctly understand the body's secret codes – an exciting task!

What Do You Think of When You Hear the Word "Fertility?"

Some may picture a pregnant woman, birth and babies. For others the word "fertility" will bring to mind Thanksgiving Day, or perhaps the ancient goddess of fertility who ensures the continuity of life on earth, generation after generation. These examples are only the outcome of fertility; however, being fertile means being able to produce new life. For example, if we say that the land is fertile, we mean it is able to produce abundant crops. If an animal is described as fertile, it means it is able to produce new offspring.

Generally speaking, humans have fewer children now than they used to. Today a woman gives birth, on average, less than twice in a lifetime and so uses very little of all the years that she is actually fertile.

What Does This All Mean for You?

Have you experienced your first period yet? If so, did anyone tell you that it is now possible for you to have children? At the moment that's probably not important to you. Perhaps you

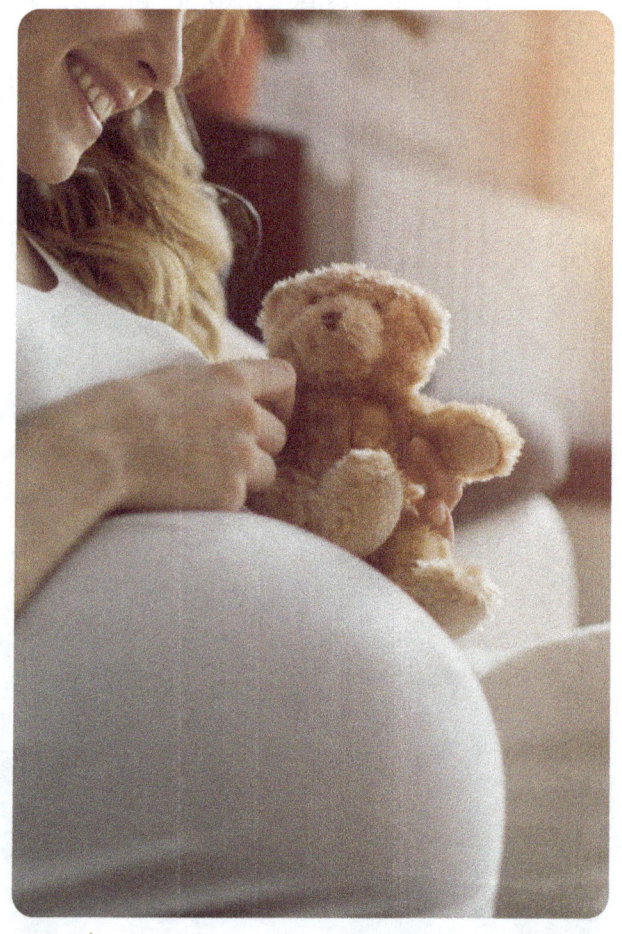

Usually you think of a pregnant woman when you hear the word "fertility."

think that it would be more practical if you could simply download this "fertility" for use at some later point in life. One click of the mouse, and "you're fertile!" Then after the baby arrives, you could click it off again.

That's simply not possible. The changes within the female body at puberty enable us to become fertile and therefore able to give birth. This amazing ability is part of being a woman, part of who you are just like breathing, walking, thinking, and loving, and it will be part of you for around 35 to 40 years, whether you have a child or not. Some women may see fertility as a burden, yet for others who desperately wish for a child, it can be a huge, unattainable goal. Many of the changes that take place at puberty in a girl's body, mind and heart are intimately connected with this gift of fertility.

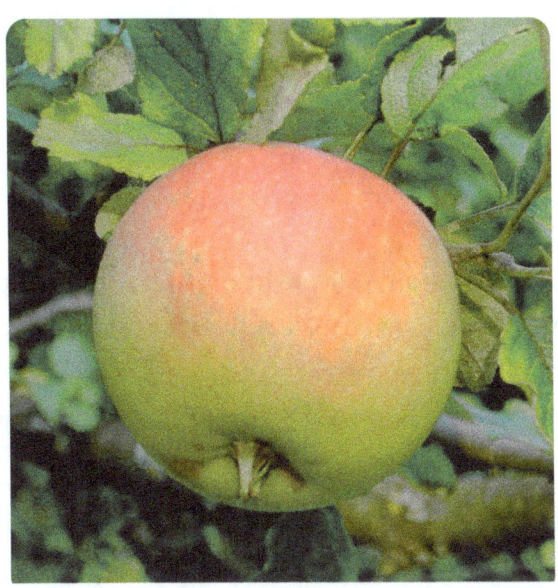

Fertility is a part of a woman's life; like breathing, walking, thinking, and loving.

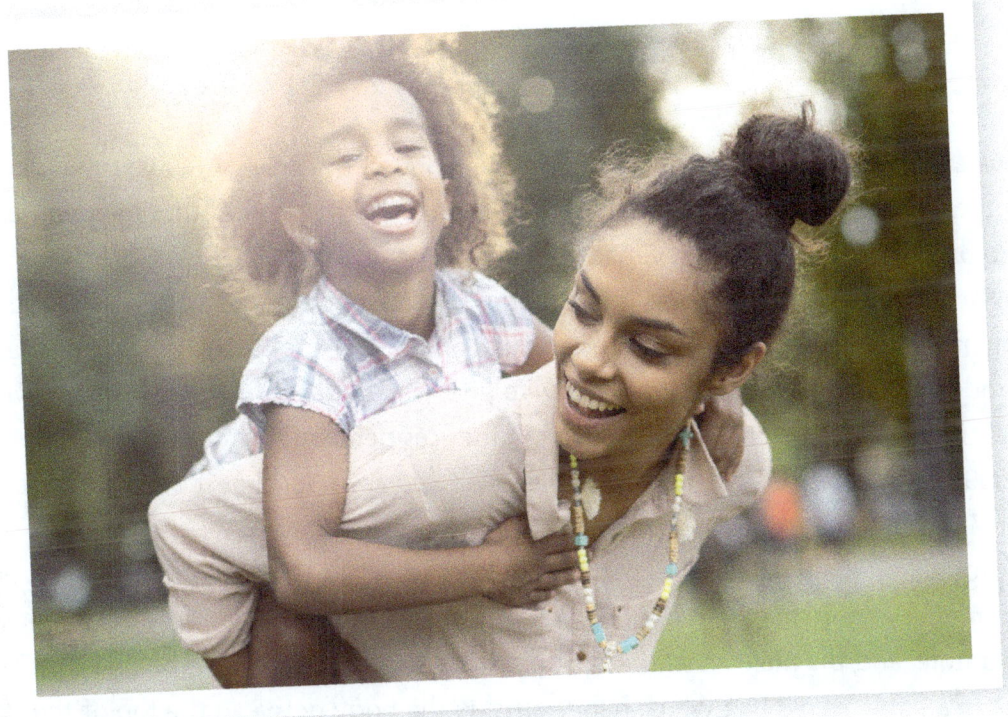

2 The Equation of Life
Sperm + Egg = Baby

For many years, folklore held that babies were brought by the stork and dropped into the households of hopeful parents. Nowadays it's common knowledge that new life is created when a man's sperm joins with a woman's egg. Sperm + Egg = Baby. Simple mathematics really! Yet this simple mathematical equation happens to be the most important equation in our lives, without it none of us would even exist. We call it **the Equation of Life!**

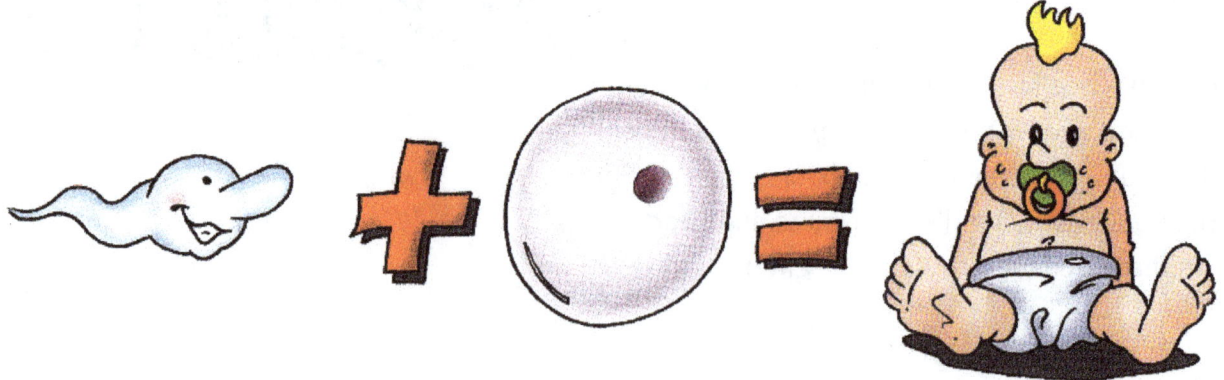

Sperm – 1,000 per Second!

Do you have a baby brother or a small cousin, maybe who can't walk yet? Do you think he already has sperm in his two tiny testicles? These little boys have many years until that happens, as males only start to produce sperm when they reach puberty.

You might be wondering where sperm are made. The male body has two testicles, and within these sperm are created. The testicles produce a huge amount of sperm and are one of the most amazing production centers in the human body. To give you an idea of just how impressive the testicles are, try to guess how many sperm a man produces per second. You won't believe the answer: 1,000 sperm every second! It's incredible when you consider that it only took one single sperm to create you.

Sperm production is a highly skilled process and it is vital that the temperature is exactly right. The optimum temperature for the production of strong, healthy sperm is a few degrees lower than body temperature, and the male anatomy is wonderfully designed to accommodate this. The two testicles rest in a skin-covered bag which hangs outside the body between the top of the thighs, called the scrotum. As the scrotum is located externally, the testicles are kept slightly cooler than the rest of the body. There is some flexibility to control the temperature further because of the use of small muscles in the scrotum. These tiny muscles are designed to pull the testicles up closer to the body to keep warm if the outside temperature is cold, for instance, when swimming in cool water. They also stretch so that the testicles can hang further away from the body,, if they need to be a bit cooler. The production zone is composed of tiny tubes called seminiferous tubules. They are arranged within the testicles in the shape of a fan, thus allowing the largest possible production area to be formed. If you were able to stretch all the tubules into one big line it would be around 1640 feet long!

Once the sperm have been created they move to the epididymis, a male has one of these located around the back of each of his two testicles. The epididymis is like a training camp for the sperm, who are like special agents. Here they mature and prepare for their mission. Only the best will survive! There is a temporary storage area for sperm in the lower part of the epididymis, here they wait for the final call to action. Every sperm takes up to three months to be fully matured.

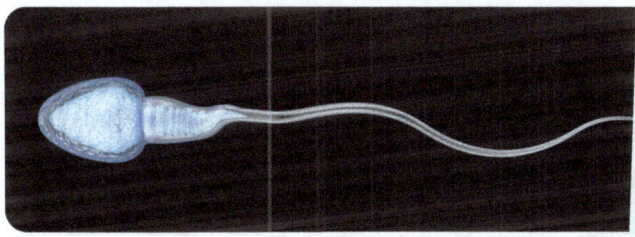

FACT
You need a factory in prime condition to make healthy sperm, so it is important that a man looks after his body. Smoking, a bad die and an unhealthy lifestyle will all affect the production of the sperm agents, which need to be in tip top shape in order to endure the journey that lies ahead.

The Sperm: Small but Impressive!

Try to imagine how big a single sperm is. Take 1/32 of an inch and divide it into 100 parts, put six of these parts back together again and you have the size of a sperm. It's so small it can only be seen under a microscope.

The sperm is made up of three different parts: the head, the middle, and the tail. The head contains the genetic information known as the chromosomes, which is half of the "building plan" required to make a baby. There is a cap on the head called the acrosome, this is made up of chemicals called enzymes which help the sperm to break into the cover of the egg. The mitochondria are located in the middle part of the sperm, and are the batteries which power the tail.

You might be wondering what happens to all the sperm that are made. Regardless of how tiny they are, if 1,000 new sperm are made every second then that's a lot of sperm! Sperm actually only last a few weeks, those that are not sent on a mission will die and be reabsorbed by the body.

The Equation of Life

When the final call comes from the brain, the sperm are released to start their journey. The adventure has begun, the mission has started, and there is no return! The agents travel together in vast numbers along a tube known as the vas deferens. In comparison to the tiny seminiferous tubules, the vas is like a huge motorway.

> **FACT**
> The vas takes the sperm from the testicles up into the pelvis. Each vas is about 1 foot long – and the width of a piece of spaghetti or thin red licorice.

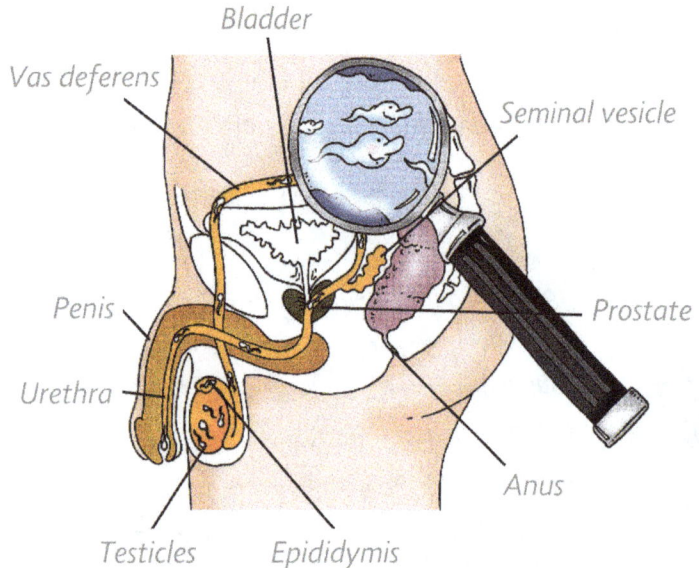

The male fertility organs.

The agents use a huge amount of energy on their journey and are grateful when they reach the seminal vesicles, which provide fructose enriched fluid for energy and vitamin C. The agents swim on and on, until they reach a gate in their path called the prostate. Measuring about the size of a walnut, the prostate is an important area in a man's pelvis as it is here the vas meets the urethra, marking the final part of the sperm's journey in the male body. The urethra is also the tube that carries urine from the bladder to the outside. As sperm cannot survive in urine, it is important that there is a gate in the prostate that stops the sperm and the urine from mixing.

Another important job the prostate has is to add special fluid for the agents to swim in; this prostate fluid combines with the sperm and forms seminal fluid. To complete the mission, the sperm travel along the urethra, which is in the penis, and must leave the male body to reach the Queen Egg. You will find out how the adventurous journey continues in Chapter 3.

105 year-old man has just become the father of a healthy baby girl. He had difficulties when he tried to register his new-born baby. The registrars considered it to be impossible for a man of his age to father a child. It was only possible to prove he was actually the father after a blood test.

From Puberty up until Old Age: Ready at Any Time?

Do you think this newspaper cutting is real, or is someone telling a joke? This is actually possible. A man is capable of making his contribution to creating a child right from the very first ejaculation, which a boy normally experiences between the ages of 9 and 14, up until the very last. In providing sperm, the man has completed his part in the Equation of Life.

The Egg – Rare and Precious

The situation is completely different in the case of women's fertility. The egg provided by your body for the creation of new life is a miracle.

Simply the Biggest!

Of all the cells in the human body, the egg is the largest. It's so big that it is just about visible to the naked eye.

Prick a hole in a piece of paper with a small, sharp needle. This gives you a good idea of the size of a fully grown egg.

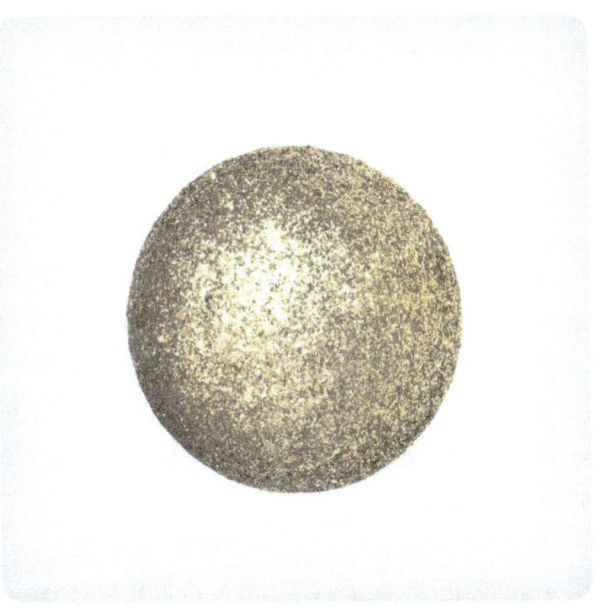

The egg – rare and precious like a golden ball.

All Eggs in Place since Birth

In contrast to men, women are born with all their eggs already in their body. The two ovaries are like small treasure chests storing the eggs since birth. When a girl reaches puberty, there will be about 400,000 eggs available. That's quite a lot, when you consider that all we need is one single egg to create a new life. The interesting thing is that the eggs age with us; for example, if you are twelve years old, your eggs are also twelve years old. A fifty year old woman's eggs will have been around for the same amount of years she has. It's therefore understandable that a woman will at some stage reach menopause, also referred to as the "change of life." Menopause occurs not because a woman has run out of eggs, but the fact that the few remaining are too tired for a great adventure.

Up until puberty it's almost as if the eggs are in hibernation. As soon as puberty begins, a group of about 20-25 eggs are then woken up at regular intervals. Only one of these eggs will become the chosen "Queen Egg" and be allowed to grow further, mature, and eventually leave the ovary in a process called ovulation. Ovulation takes place roughly 400 times during the fertile stage of a woman's life.

The Eggs' Performance: Short but Spectacular

The egg is the cell in the human body with the shortest lifespan. The nerve cells or the heart muscle cells have to hold out for a lifetime, but an egg doesn't survive much longer than a half a day once ovulation has happened and it has left the ovary. This short period of time, 12 to 18 hours to be precise, is the only chance for the egg to meet a sperm.

Preparations for a Special Guest

Imagine you have just arrived home from school. It's around 4pm when your telephone starts to ring. You can hardly believe it, on the other end of the line you hear the manager of your favorite female pop star! He says: "Congratulations! You are one of only 10 girls who have been chosen. If you are really lucky, tonight at 7pm your door bell might ring and when you open the door there will be your favorite pop star standing on your doorstep. She wants to visit you and may even want to stay overnight!"

What would you do now? Once you've overcome the initial shock, you'd probably call or text your best friends. They'd want to be in on everything and promise to help you with all the necessary preparations. Together you'd tidy up your home and make sure there are plenty of delicious things to eat and drink. You might even decide to hire a caterer as such a special guest needs to be looked after exceptionally well.

How do you think this story could end? It's unlikely that your pop star will come. Occasionally people do hit the jackpot and win the first prize of a car or a vacation. But this does not happen often, and even more rarely to us. If the manager were to

> **SHAYNA (14)**
> It's a strange thing with this menstrual cycle. I'm not sure what to make of it. I'd be so frustrated if all my work turned out to be a waste of time. Our teacher said that in the man's case, it's even more extreme. Millions, or was it billions, of sperm are produced in vain. But the body appears to have little problem with that. Everything is supplied in abundance, over and over again without considering whether there's any point to it or not.

tell us that we weren't lucky this time, then we'd make the best of it, simply have a party anyway and then clean everything up. Now if a weeks later the manager called you to say yet again your pop star is coming to visit, would you still make such a huge effort?

So what does this story have to do with your body? A great deal actually! Your body also receives a wonderful message again and again that perhaps a "Special Guest" will visit, that the Equation of Life (a baby) could become reality. Our body reacts to this wonderful opportunity and immediately begins to prepare itself with the help of many friends which you will meet later. It even has its own sort of catering service. If this Special Guest doesn't arrive, then everything is quickly cleaned up so the body can prepare for a new visitor all over again.

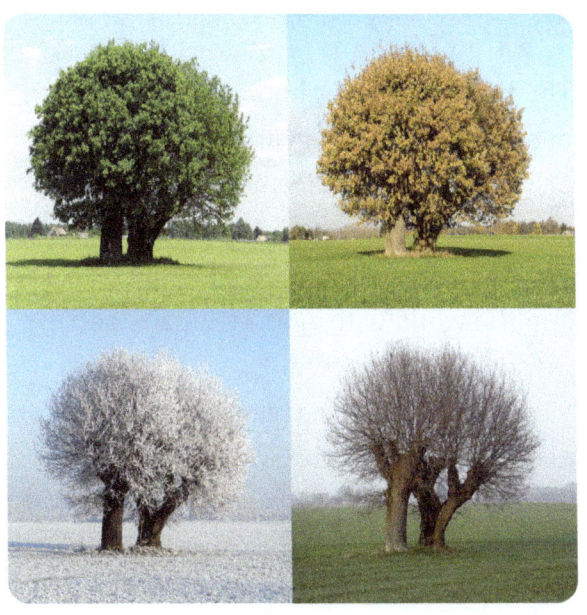

A woman's cycle is a reflection of nature's seasons.

Women's Menstrual Cycle: A Reflection of Nature

For many years the task of a woman's body is to prepare for a big event, followed by a time of cleaning up. Things can often look very different on the "Stage of Life" depending on whether the preparations are still under way or if the cleaning up is in progress.

Just like a circle that has neither a beginning nor an end, these activities in a woman's body continue without effort over many years. The repetitive manner of the woman's cycle is almost like a reflection of nature. Just as the seasons change and repeat themselves over and over, the woman's body is in a constant state of renewal or replacement. Hence, this kind of loop is called a "cycle."

Nature has a lot of wealth and so does a woman's body, it does not need to conserve and can afford to supply everything in abundance each, and every time.

On the Stage of Life

The "Stage of Life" lies deep inside the female's body: below the belly button, protected by the pelvic bones, nestled between the abdominal wall, the bladder and the bowel. It consists of the ovaries, the uterus with the fallopian tubes, and the vagina.

The Two Treasure Chests – the Ovaries

The two ovaries are about as big as walnuts or small plums and are attached to the pelvic wall by small ligaments. There are great treasures hidden in the ovaries: around 400,000 eggs, which every little girl comes into the world with, and a woman's best friends, the estrogens.

> **FACT**
> *Estrogen and progesterone are female hormones, messenger substances that are generated in the ovaries and find their way from there through the bloodstream all over the body.*

Day and night the female hormones work as messengers, helping with preparations throughout the woman's body to ensure she feels well. The final treasure is an excellent catering service called progesterone. Just like estrogen, progesterone also supports the woman with all the necessary preparations that take place time and again during her cycle. We'll soon be hearing quite a lot about these excellent companions: the "Estrogen Friends" and the "Progesterone Team."

A Luxury Hotel for the Baby – the Uterus

The uterus, also known as the womb, lies in the middle of the pelvis. It provides the hotel that the baby moves into for nine months. At first sight, this accommodation may appear to be a somewhat strange construction, but upon closer examination it proves to be extremely practical. The hotel resembles the shape of a pear, measuring 2-3 inches, with the thicker end at the top. Instead of the hard, unyielding brick walls usually used for a house, the outer walls of the uterus consist of a soft flexible layer of muscle. This ingenious invention provides a small space in its empty state, but should a little guest decide to make him or herself at home there, it can be developed into a spacious Luxury Suite. When the guest finally leaves his lodgings after nine months, this amazing muscular construction manages to shrink itself again. The muscles contract during labor to push the baby out of the door!

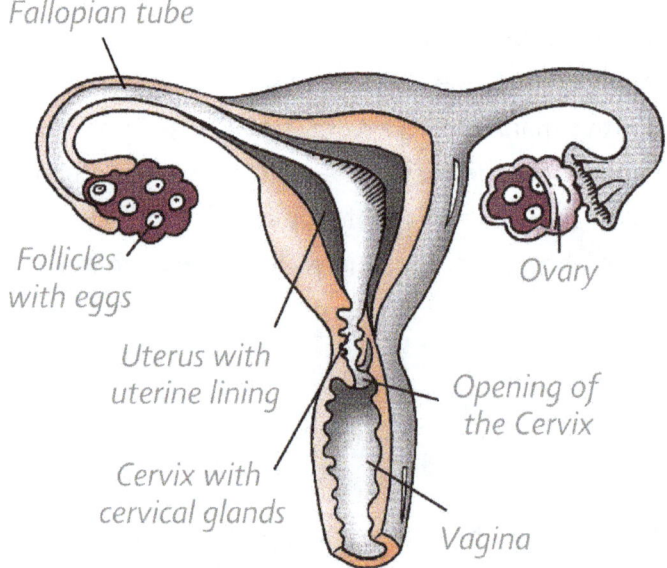

The female sexual organs – The Stage of Life in a woman's body.

The Good Life – Cozy Corners in the Uterine Lining

The Luxury Suite is very comfortable and child-friendly. Cozy corners are lovingly created in the top layer of the uterine lining. If a guest has an all inclusive reservation, he is well provided for in the form of nutrients, oxygen, intimate body contact with Mom, and (at least at the beginning!) lots of space to move.

Just as one would expect in a five star hotel, each new guest gets fresh luxuries: a fresh bed, flowers, and food. To make this possible the top layer of the uterine lining must first be disposed of, which happens with menstrual bleeding.

The Journey of the Egg through the Fallopian Tube

At the top end of the pear-shaped uterus, there are tunnels to the left and right which are called the fallopian tubes. They are the connection between the uterus and the ovaries and provide the meeting place for the egg and the sperm. When the egg is ripe and ready to start its great adventure, the finger-shaped ends of the fallopian tube are led, as if by magic, to exactly the right point of the ovary to catch the egg as it bursts out.

If by chance any sperm are around at this moment, fertilization may take place here in the outer tunnel section of the fallopian tube, with the union of egg and sperm.

The fallopian tube now transports the small embryo to its hotel room. Measuring only .04-.08 inches in diameter, the tunnel tube is very narrow. So for this reason there is a type of conveyor belt system in place. As if being carried along by gentle waves, this new life is rolled forward in the direction of the uterus with the help of little microscopic hairs known as cilia.

> **FACT**
> The uterine lining is made up of two layers. Only the top layer changes during the course of the menstrual cycle. It is replaced each time after it bleeds out of the womb during a period.

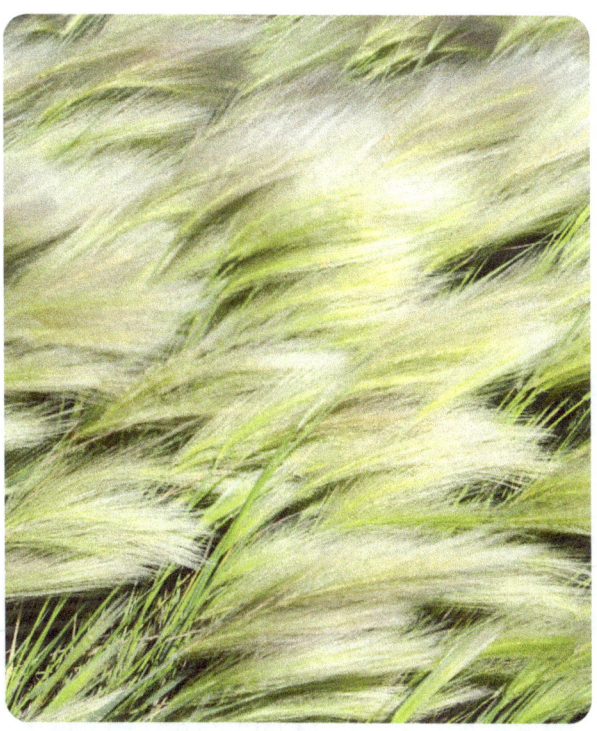

Similar to this feather grass the cilia in the fallopian tube sway in the direction of the uterus, moving the fertilized egg as if being carried by gentle waves.

Gym and Wellness Center in the Cervix

The lower, narrower part of the pear shaped uterus is known as the neck of the uterus and is called the cervix; it has a canal inside and fulfills different tasks than the hotel above. On the sides of the canal are entries to about 100 glands, these are the gym and wellness center for travelling sperm, but we'll get back to discussing them later. The canal leads to the lower opening of the cervix, the "Gate of Life", which then extends into the vagina.

The Entrance Hall Leading to the Stage of Life – The Vagina

This elastic tube of muscle, which is roughly 4 inches in length, is known as the vagina and creates the connection between the uterus and the outside world. The vagina is the most important entrance hall as many events take place here. Menstrual bleeding, which is the result of the monthly renewal and replacement work on the Luxury Suite, flows out of the body through the vagina. The vagina can also receive and embrace the man's penis, it is here where the sperm are released during ejaculation. The baby must also push through this canal upon leaving its luxury hotel after nine months, by then the vagina will be so elastic and stretchy that the baby's head will fit through.

Protection for the Vagina – The Hymen

The Stage of Life is protected in several ways. From the outside, the entrance into the vagina is covered by the inner and outer lips of the vulva: the labia. They grow during puberty, are very different in size and are darker in color in adult women. At the entrance to the vagina most young girls have a thin skin covering known as the hymen, which varies in thickness and flexibility from one girl to another. The hymen can also sometimes be quite soft, or it may not be there at all. One of the tasks of the hymen is to protect the Stage of Life during childhood. Through the remaining opening the menstrual blood can still flow without any problems. During puberty the hymen becomes wider and looser, and is stretched by using tampons or during sexual intercourse. Sometimes it may tear slightly and can bleed a little, but not always.

> **KATIE (12)**
> We were going over the topic of the female reproductive organs in school. The boys were really making fun of us. If they hadn't been present, I might have had the nerve to ask about the hymen, but with them there – no way, it was totally humiliating!

3 The Equation of Life
How a New Life Begins

The woman's Stage of Life has now been described and some of the main stars, the sperm and egg, have been introduced. So now the show can start! One at a time though, so first up on stage are the sperm.

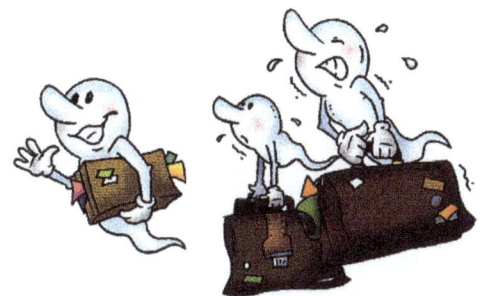

Do you know how many sperm enter the vagina during ejaculation? 1,000? 10,000? 100,000? Maybe even a million? Unbelievably 200-700 million sperm are sent on their way to try their luck. What awaits the sperm inside the vagina? And how do they get to the ultimate finish line, the egg?

The Adventurous Journey of the Sperm

Good times – Bad times
A woman's body is not very gentle with the sperm, but this is with good reason. A woman's body has a direct path from the outside to the abdomen, via the vagina, uterus, fallopian tubes and ovaries. To prevent infection from entering, the vagina has a special protective mechanism to fight off bacteria and other invaders. The vagina has an acidic environment which the sperm don't like very much.

Escaping to the Frontline?
The sperm don't want to stay in the vagina; they want to continue on towards the egg. To do this, they have to reach the top of the vagina and pass through the cervix into the uterus. The sperm meet even more obstacles here as the Gate of Life is closed. A thick, sticky plug of mucus blocks the entrance to the uterus. Some of the stronger sperm may try to penetrate the plug and will regret this as they find themselves in a thick and dense mesh. The sperm will quickly get stuck, their heads are too big and the mesh gets tighter and tighter. During most of the woman's cycle the sperm will die in the vagina within 30 minutes to three hours, their adventure is over before it even started!

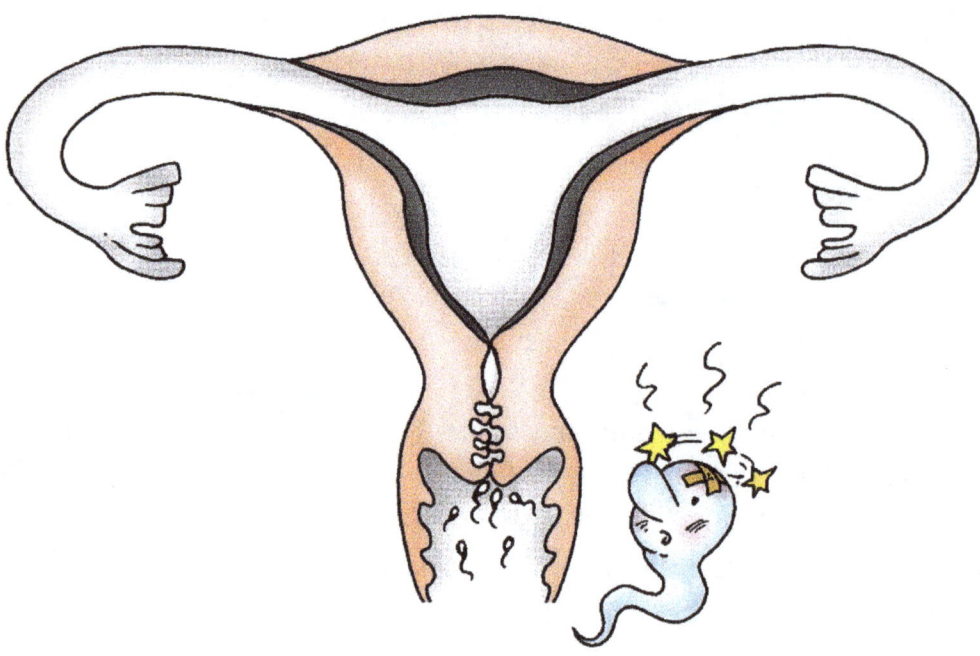

During most of the woman's cycle the sperm will die within thirty minutes to three hours.

When the Timing is Right – Full Speed Ahead!

But there are also more fortunate sperm, the ones who have good timing!

The circumstances aren't always this bad, and the climate is not always this rough. When a woman's body begins to prepare for the Equation of Life to become a reality, the situation changes. For a few days, the Gate of Life opens. At first it only opens a tiny bit, then a little more, and still some more until it is .3 inches (0.75cm) open. To the sperm, it looks like the door has been flung open and a welcome mat put out! Something else has happened, the mucus plug has dissolved and a liquid is flowing from the uterus. The sperm, which looked like they would die in the vagina, are drawn towards it and quickly realize it's the lifeline they so desperately need! It is as if the female body has produced a "Magic Potion" for the sperm, but this only happens for a few days.

This Magic Potion is called cervical mucus, and the hungry sperm take in vital nutrients from it, including essential sugar. With each passing second, they gain new strength and energy, but that alone still isn't enough!

> **FACT**
>
> *In the vagina, sperm die within 30 minutes to three hours.*

On the Way to the Leisure Center

Like deep sea divers, the sperm dive into the Magic Potion and can now move weightlessly. The cervical mucus contains wide channels, and within these, sperm are moved forward like cars on a highway. So in a few minutes the sperm escape from the vagina and into the cervix, where it gets even better! On either side of the highway are many exits called the cervical crypts, and just like a gas or service station, these crypts provide refreshment and a place to rest.

According to the latest research, when the cervix is open and cervical mucus is present, some of the sperm are sucked up into the uterus. Covered and protected by nutritional cervical mucus, sperm are moved swiftly upwards to the opening of the fallopian tube, which leads to the egg.

> **FACT**
>
> The cervical mucus has many functions. It nourishes the sperm, gives them energy and protects them from the acidic environment in the vagina. The mucus channels the sperm up the reproductive tract and filters out the unhealthy sperm so only the best get ahead.

The sperm that are left behind get the chance to enjoy the pleasures of the cervical crypts for longer, and they can chill for a while in the cervical mucus.

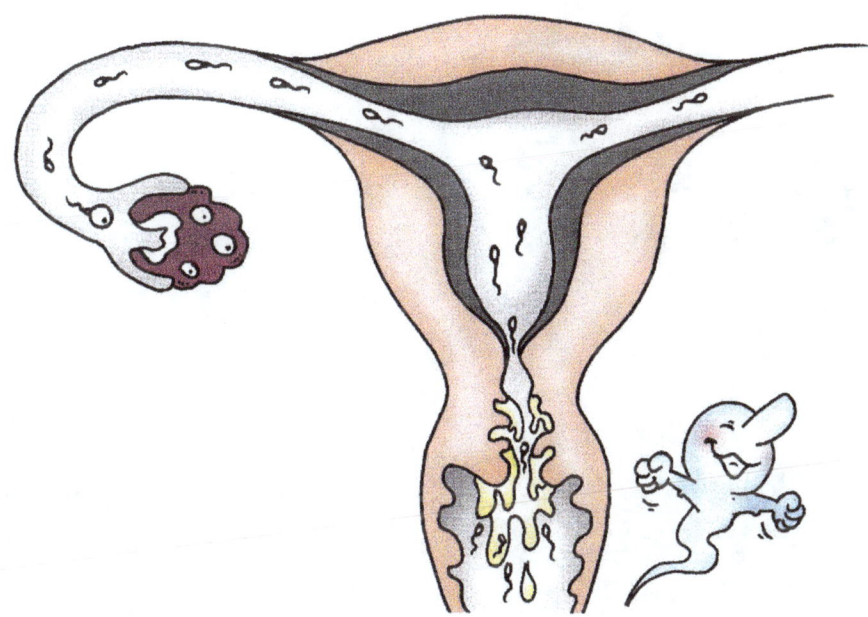

During a few days of the cycle, the cervical mucus runs into the vagina and the sperm can survive in the cervical crypts for the next 3 to 5 days.

Now the Fun Starts…
Leisure Time for Sperm

The cervical mucus is a great product but is only available for a few days. It is produced by about 100 glands in the cervix, exclusively for sperm. In the "Leisure Center" (spa) of the cervix, the sperm are spoiled; they can eat, drink, and prepare. Some sperm stay a short time, others longer; it can be from two to five days. Strengthened and full of the spirit of adventure, they will carry on with their travels.

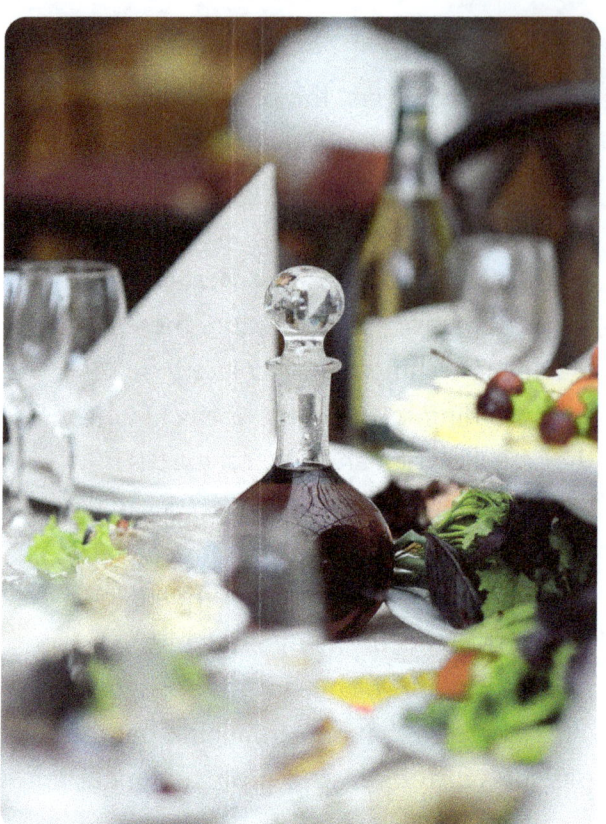

Sperm enjoy the cervical mucus in the cervical glands like we would a gourmet meal.

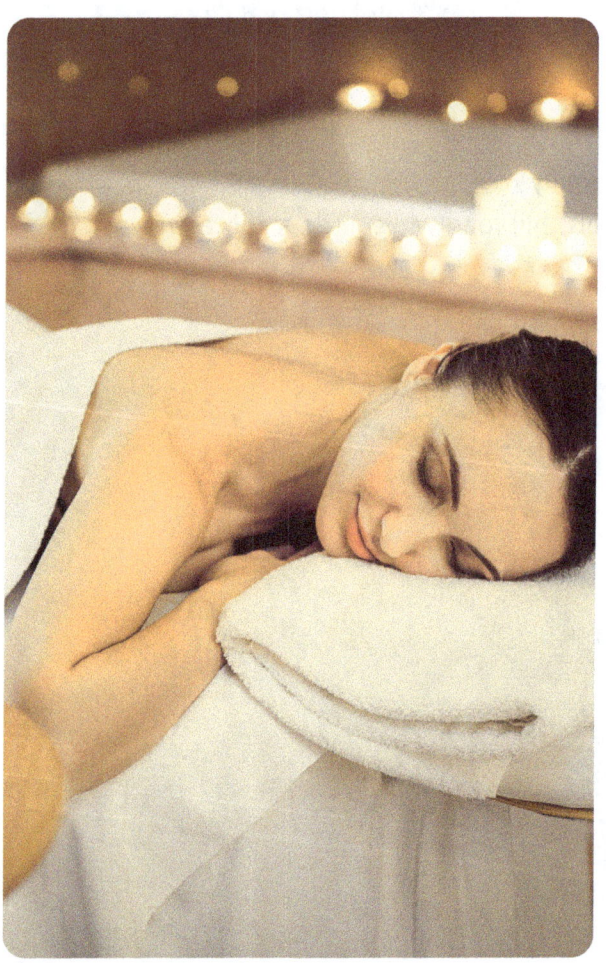

Sperm can treat themselves in the cervix, like people do in a spa.

> **FACT**
> *Sperm can live up to five days in the cervical mucus.*

Right or Left: Where will the Egg be?

Initially the path leads the sperm through the dark cave of the uterus. At the top of the uterus, on the left and right, lie the entrances to the ovaries. Which way should they go? Good question.

If it was known in which ovary the egg was

growing, then where ovulation was happening would also be know. But nature keeps that a secret! There is no certain pattern, as the chances of going left or right are the same in each cycle: 50/50. Only the sperm that choose the correct fallopian tube get the chance to win the jackpot: the egg.

The latest research suggests that in order to increase the sperm's chance of finding the egg, the female body again gives them some assistance. Tiny muscles at the entrance of the fallopian tube contract rhythmically, causing the sperm to be sucked up and led to the ovary containing the maturing egg.

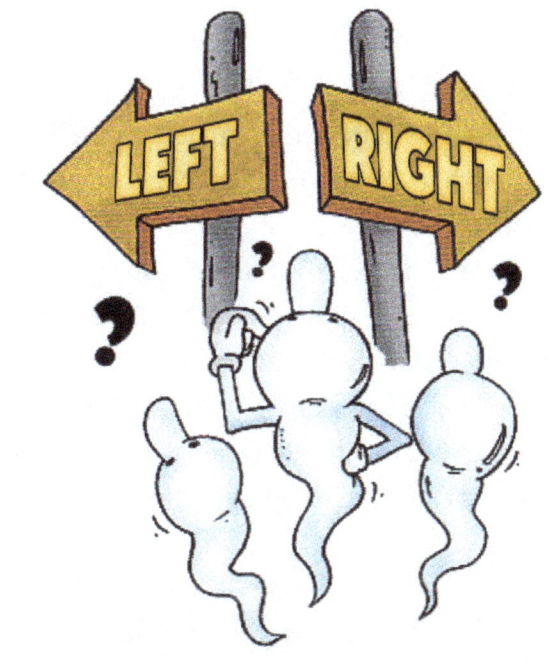

The Final Hurdle!

On the last part of the journey the sperm will, once more, have a difficult task. Without the support of the Magic Potion, the sperm's energy stores start to dwindle, and they now have to swim against the flow in the fallopian tubes as the cilia try to move them back towards the uterus. And so the selection of sperm continues. Many die after being trapped in the deep folds of the uterus, getting stuck in ravines, while others will be attacked by the body's police force (white cells) and get no further. Some sperm will get too tired and give up. From the millions that start the journey, only a few manage to get to the end of the fallopian tube, where an egg is likely to be waiting. There are only a few hundred sperm left that are ready for the last hurdle, but now teamwork is required. The effort of every sperm is important as they work in accordance to the motto: "All for one and one for all!" Together they must now use their acrosome cap to break down the shell of the egg.

> **FACT**
> There is a theory that the egg herself chooses the sperm she lets in.

Whether you call it luck, fate, or destiny, it is not the first or the quickest sperm that wins the prize. It is the sperm that ends up in the right place at the right time, the one closest to where the first opening appears in the shell.

The excitement is high as only one can win! What happens next is the most exciting occurrence in the story of our world. The start of a new life!

And the Winner is…Fertilization

There is now only one sperm left on the Stage of Life, with its own extraordinary genetic code. This sperm is the winner!

When the head of this lucky sperm enters the egg, something special happens. An automatic security system is activated by a chemical signal. In the blink of an eye, everything is locked. Once one sperm is in, no other sperm can enter, and again, the body acts with good reason. A healthy

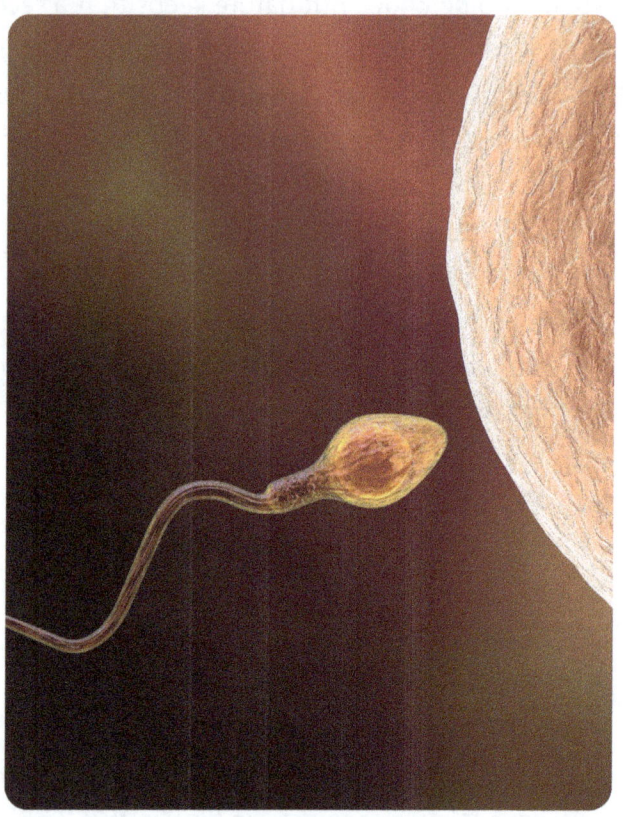

Is that the winner? A sperm on its way into an egg.

human only has a certain number of genes, half from its mother and half from its father. As soon as the sperm is in, the tail stops moving and falls off. The important bit now is the head, with its tiny nucleus. This contains all the information and genetic codes that the father passes to his child for life.

Boy or Girl?

The sex of the child is determined by the father. An X chromosome in the sperm creates a girl, a Y chromosome creates a boy.

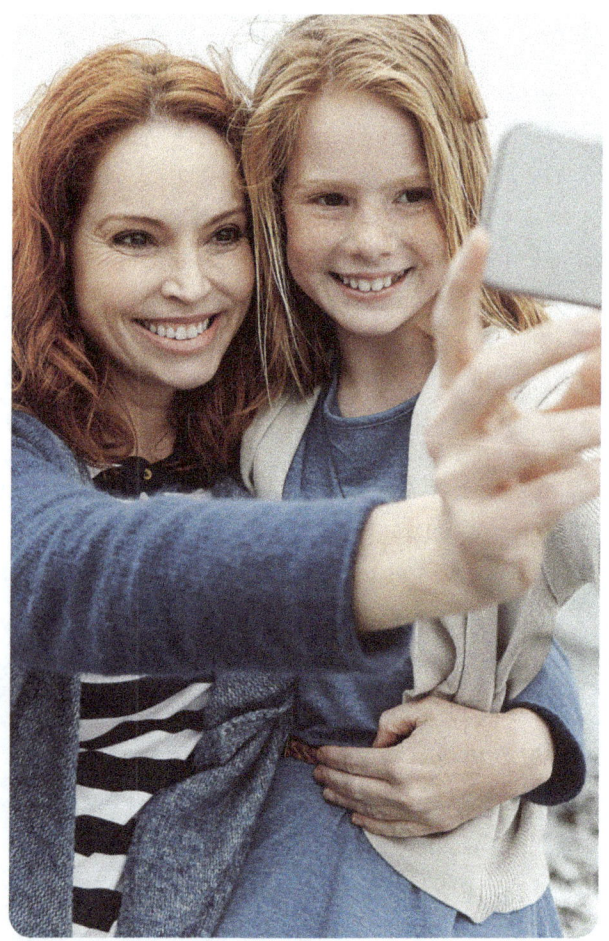

The similarities between mother and daughter are already there at conception.

You are the champion!

Have you ever thought about the moment when your life began? You, yourself were once the winning sperm – from millions! And not only this, you were also the chosen "Queen Egg"! So from the very beginning of your life, you are a double winner. You gained all the things that you are so proud of today: maybe your blue eyes, skinny legs, and math skills. You also won the things that you are not so happy with, such as your height perhaps or maybe your hair color? You are a winner with all your characteristics, whether you like them or not. Whenever life seems a bit hard, never forget this: The fact you came into being from the winning sperm and the Queen Egg is even bigger than a lottery win. You are completely unique; no one is quite like you.

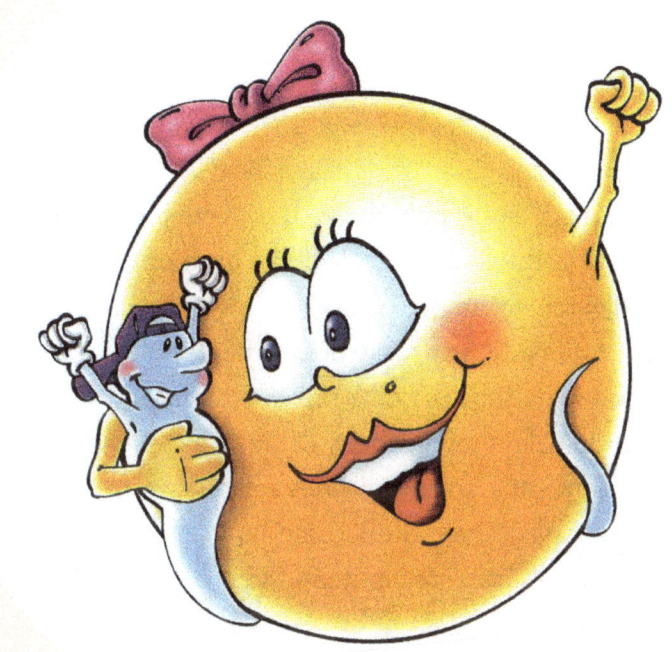

- **You are a miracle!**
- **You are unique!**
- **It is amazing to be alive!**
- **It is great that you exist!**

Inside the big egg, there is the nucleus containing the mother's genes. Soon a new human life will start. The two nuclei head toward one another, finally they merge and that's the beginning of a new, unique life! At that moment, the appearance of the new person is determined: eye and hair color, size, facial features and even certain diseases and talents!

> **FACT**
> Identical twins happen when the dividing egg gets separated on the way through the fallopian tube. Having the same building plan, they continue growing into two identical people. They will be the same sex and look the same, other people may mix them up.

Out of One, Comes Two: The Egg Divides

Fertilization is only the start of a huge growing process in the woman's body. If all goes well it will end in the "Grand Finale"; the birth of a baby. But there are still many obstacles to overcome and dangers to survive.

Already, just a few hours after fertilization, the egg divides for the first time. The cilia in the fallopian tube move the cells, now called the embryo, in the direction of the uterus. It will take four or five days to get there. During its journey the embryo divides again and again, two cells become four, four cells become eight, and so on.

No Signal during this Time

During the egg's journey through the fallopian tube, the woman's body does not yet know that a new life has begun. From the moment the egg is released at ovulation, it is floating in space and the contact between body and egg is broken. The first few days are the most dangerous. Not every embryo reaches the haven of the uterus, where preparations for its arrival are in full flow.

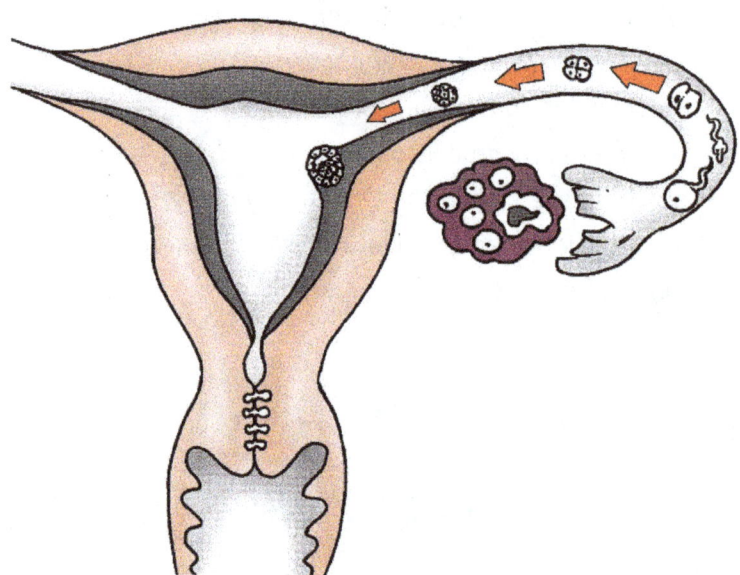

Here you can see the fertilization of the egg at the end of the fallopian tube, and the four or five day journey to the uterus. As soon as fertilization occurs, cell division starts.

Those that do manage to make it will have overcome the biggest hurdle now. When the little guest first arrives in the wide open hall of the uterine hotel, from the narrow confines of the tube, it may feel a little lost. Over the next few days it can have a good look around and choose a cozy corner to settle down in for the next nine months. A week or so after fertilization, there will be another very important moment.

Hello Mommy! I'm here!

By the time the little guest arrives in the endometrium it consists of more than 100 cells. It now makes contact with its mother's body and they grow together. A close connection between mother and child is made, which will

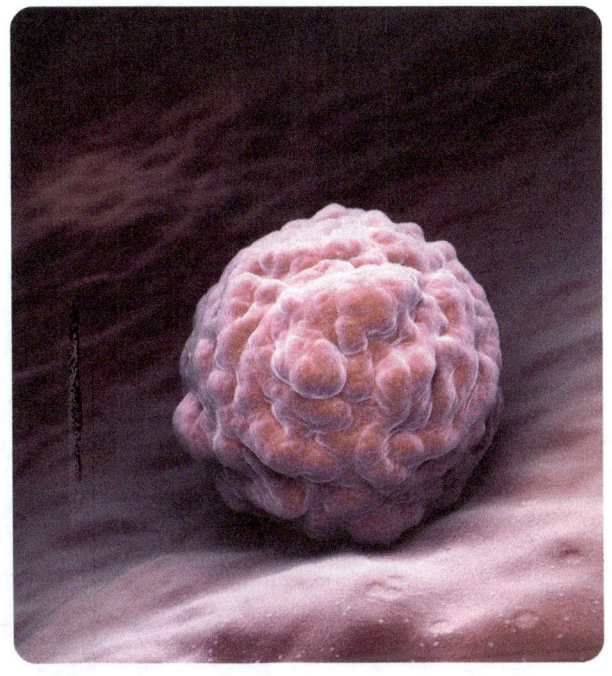

Six days after fertilization, the fertilized egg has become a blastocyst and cuddles up inside the uterus.

be the umbilical cord from which the child will receive nourishment from its mother. Before that happens the mother has to know she is carrying a baby. As soon as the connection is re-established, the child sends the very first love letter to Mommy. The first message from the child to the mother is a chemical messenger sent via the bloodstream, a hormone

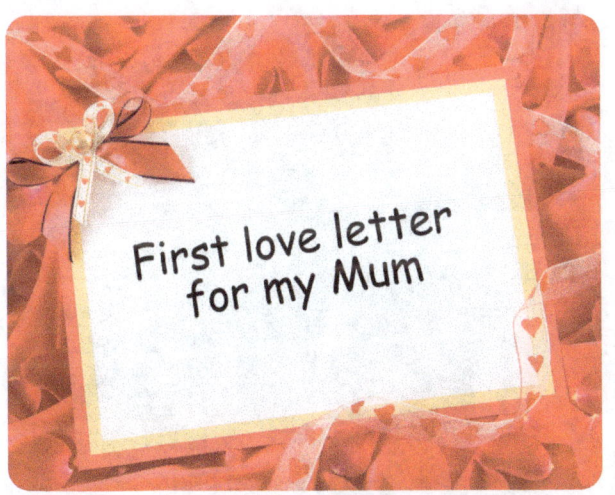

known as HCG, or human chorionic gonadotrophin. Two weeks after fertilization, the HCG hormone can be detected in the mother's urine. A pregnancy test would be positive now; the mother knows she is expecting a baby!

FACT *The nestling into the endometrium, also known as implantation, takes place about one week after ovulation and fertilization.*

The Equation of Life

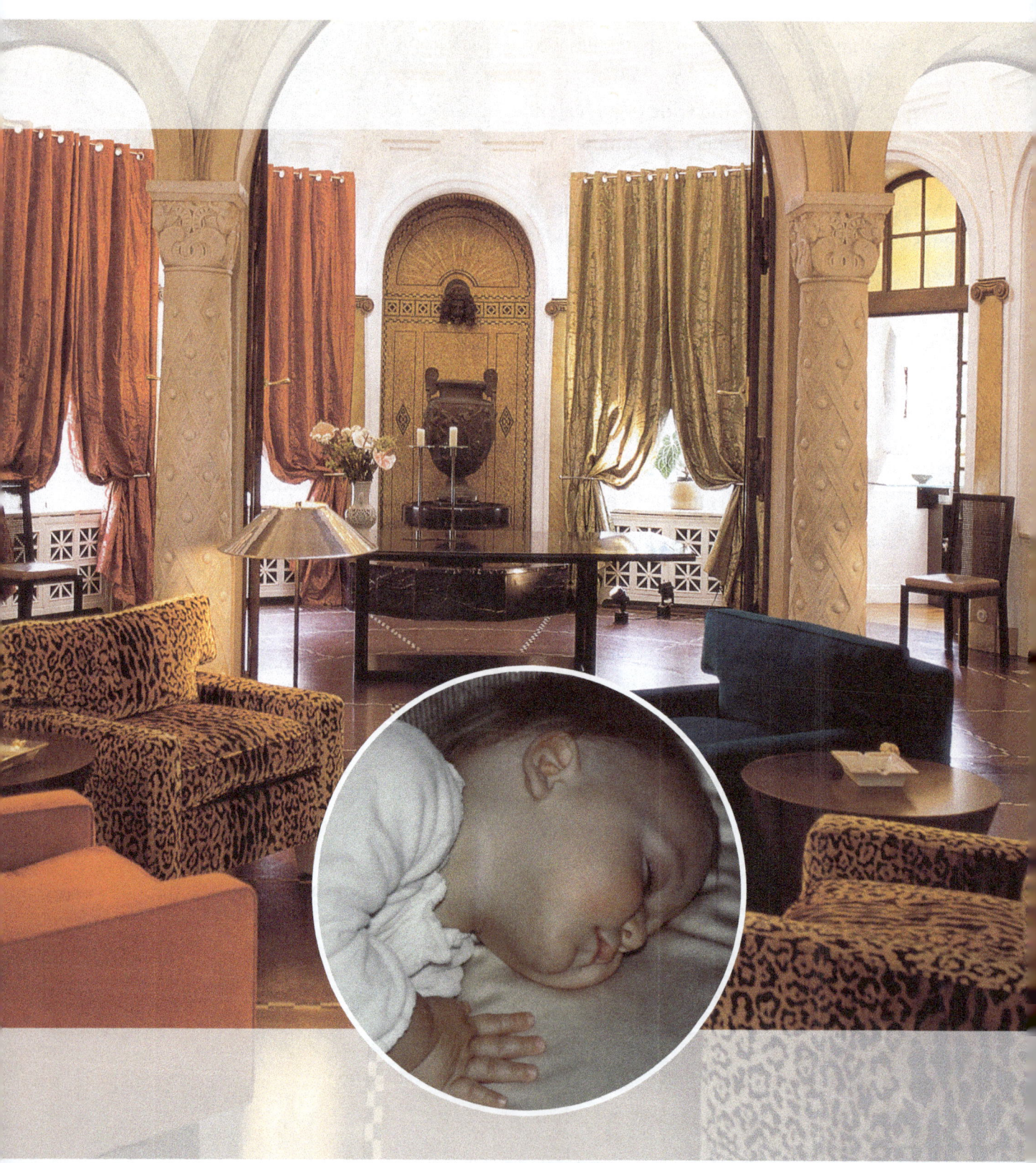

It's all about Timing – Fertile or Not Fertile?

A woman can only get pregnant if the egg, released at ovulation, is caught by the fallopian tube. It is there that the egg may meet with a sperm up to 18 hours after ovulation. As you are now aware, this is not a daily occurrence!

The life cycle of an unfertilized egg is fairly unremarkable. In a normal cycle, when the egg lands in the fallopian tube after ovulation, there is no one there to greet it. The egg will survive for a few hours and then it will slowly dissolve and vanish.

In a cycle of about 30 days, the egg will only be available to be fertilized for around 12 to18 hours; the sperm must be present at that time to stand a chance. They must have psychic abilities, surely, or otherwise the human race would be extinct by now! Or maybe there is another way. Do you remember the sperm that stopped off in the lovely cervical crypts? Thanks to the Magic Potion they enjoyed in this Leisure Center they can survive a number of days. This can only happen if the sperm arrive in the body during the days before ovulation. The sperm are gradually moved from the cervix to the fallopian tubes. This clever, gradual move by the woman's body ensures that there is still a supply of sperm at ovulation, even if they were deposited in the vagina some days before.

In optimal conditions, with the best quality cervical mucus, the healthiest sperm can survive for five days.

> **FACT**
> *Many think that the egg travels to the uterus and is flushed out with the menstrual flow. That is not true! The egg dissolves in the fallopian tube and has nothing to do with the woman's period.*

Complete the Equation of Life!
Now what was the Equation of Life again?

Sperm + Egg = Baby?

But you now know this is only partly correct. The dramatic events between the egg and sperm will only happen during the so called fertile phase, when cervical mucus is present.

The Equation of Life should really be:

(Sperm + Cervical Mucus) + Egg = Baby!

The Equation of Life

Now you can calculate how long a man and woman are fertile together by the number of days she can get pregnant: three to five days before ovulation plus the one day that the egg is viable, making a total of between four to six days. Neither man nor woman can be fertile on their own.

That's a really short time, isn't it? You will get to know how these changes in a woman's body are possible in the next chapter.

> **FACT**
> In medicine, one speaks about the "fertility triad," meaning that three factors are needed for fertility: the egg, the sperm, and the cervical mucus.

Equation of Life completed:

(Sperm + Cervical Mucus)   +   Egg   =   Baby

Three to five days   +   one day

Four to Six days of shared fertility between a man and a woman in one cycle.

4 Clear the Stage for the Cycle Show

Imagine that you're going to the theater. Before the play begins all you can see is a red curtain covering the stage. Sooner or later, the curtain opens. The stage is black and empty, but you remain seated and wait patiently. You are waiting a few weeks. Then something happens; the red curtain closes again and remains closed for a few days. This unexciting show repeats itself roughly every month for all women around the world. The red curtain represents the period of course, and the blank stage the weeks in between when nothing seems to be happening. Many women rightly wonder what all the fuss is about and why we need a period.

Of course every woman notices when she has her period, but very few have any idea what actually takes place on the Stage of Life between these periods. It is not at all surprising that for many women the monthly period is viewed as an annoyance. Some women would probably be quite glad to live without their period altogether; however, once you understand that an exciting and fascinating drama is actually taking place inside your body every month, it never needs to feel like that for you. So, let's clear the stage for the "Cycle Show!"

As we go through the Cycle Show we will compare it to a real life production at the theater. The hormones, tissues and organs in the body are described and given names like actors, with the play taking place on the Stage of Life that is your body. The comparison of a woman's cycle to a show at a theater will hopefully help you to remember the information.

The Control Center – The Brain Regulates Hormones

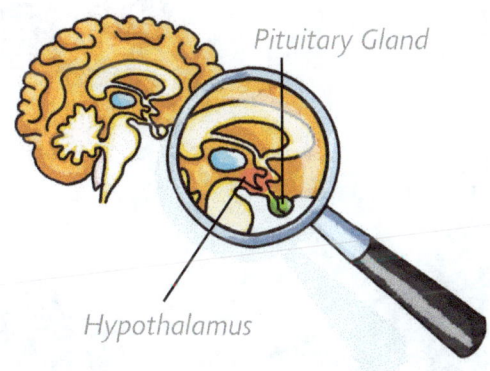

Our brain is the chief fertility organ. All directions stem from here in the hypothalamus and in the pituitary gland.

You are already familiar with the Stage of Life in the woman's pelvis. The ovaries, fallopian tubes, uterus, and vagina are all locations for exciting events, but the Cycle Show doesn't just take place there. The stage directions come from somewhere completely different; the human brain.

First Act of the Cycle Show – The Estrogens Start Working

The Cycle Show officially begins on the very first day of menstruation. The top layer of the uterine lining dissolves and blood leaks out of many tiny veins. While the bleeding continues, a message is sent by the managers in the brain to tell the body that a fantastic guest, a new life, might arrive and that preparations quickly need to be made. What does this mean? Eggs have to be woken up, and if sperm arrive they need permission to enter.

Just like the first bloom of flowers after winter tell us the seasons are changing, the managers in the brain send what we can call the first "Messengers of Spring" via the bloodstream to both ovaries. They are known as FSH (follicle stimulating hormone) and they deliver the message: "Wake up, little eggs! It's time to come to life!"

The Eggs are Woken Up

As a result of these messages, about 20 to 25 tiny eggs are woken out of their hibernation and start to grow. As the eggs are delicate and in need of protection, a liquid filled bubble, known as a follicle, grows around them, allowing them to continue to develop in the ovaries without any disturbance.

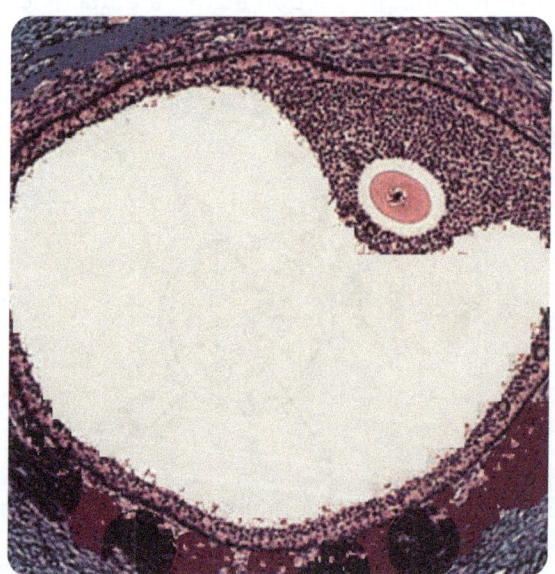

The egg grows inside a bubble called the follicle, which is filled with fluid.

The Estrogens: A Woman's Best Friends

The protective cover of a follicle is of great importance. The body does exactly the same as you would when you need help - it asks for help from friends. The eggs are woken up when the message arrives that the Equation of Life may become a reality, and this is the moment for our bodies' best friends to appear on the scene: the "Estrogen Friends." These messenger hormones develop on the cover around the egg and are the best friends a woman could ever wish for. The Estrogen Friends are extremely friendly, committed, skilled workers with artistic talent, and always ready to lend a hand. As all good friends do, they don't wait around to be asked to help. Instead they separate themselves from the follicle and spread throughout the body so that preparations can begin.

The Queen is Chosen

Meanwhile back in the ovary, a secret vote has taken place. Normally only one single egg is chosen from the many that were woken up. This selected "Queen Egg" will get bigger, and have the chance to partake in a great adventure in the process of creating new life. If you are wondering why so many eggs get woken up, it's so the body always has a choice and can therefore ensure it selects the best egg!

> **FACT**
> *How exactly one particular egg out of 20 to 25 is singled out and selected remains one of nature's secrets. When it comes to non-identical twins, something pretty special happens. Suddenly there are two eggs, equally mature and equally developed. The body can't decide which one to choose, so it says to itself: "OK, let's make an exception. This time we will have two queens!"*

All the other ripened eggs have fulfilled their role now, so they leave the stage and dissolve. The follicle containing the Queen Egg now grows bigger every day. The larger the egg becomes, the more Estrogen Friends develop on its protective cover. These best friends swarm out from the follicle via the bloodstream in order to help with preparations on the Stage of Life.

Uterine Hotel: Structural Work Begins in the Luxury Suites

At the beginning of the cycle, the top layer of the uterine lining has bled from the womb during menstruation. Several days later the Estrogen Friends bring the good news that an egg will soon be mature, and, all being well, will take the adventurous leap known as ovulation. This means there is a chance, once again, that a Special Guest may settle into the luxurious uterine hotel. The Estrogen Friends are in charge and get to work immediately; the top layer of the uterine lining is reconstructed, walls and ceilings are added, windows fitted and floors are laid. In this way, the foundations for the luxury hotel are completed.

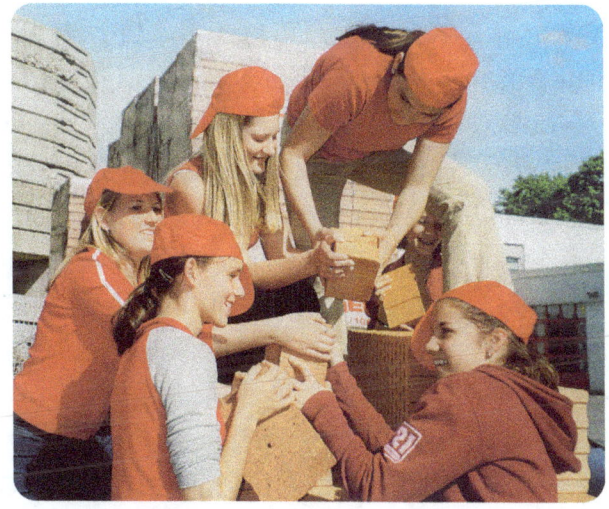

The estrogens prepare the foundation of the Luxury Hotel. The top layer of the uterine lining, that leaves the body as the monthly period, is reconstructed.

Cervix: Production of the Magic Potion Begins

If the Equation of Life is to become a reality and a new human being is to be created, then not only does the egg have to ripen, but the sperm must also be allowed to enter the scene.

As soon as the estrogens reach the cervix, they put an end to the peace and quiet there, and a new season is opened in the Leisure Center. First of all, the thick mucus plug at the cervix is removed, and then the production of the Magic Potion begins. The more estrogens that arrive there, the more intensive the preparations for the health and leisure program. The quality of the cervical mucus, which was quite concentrated, sticky, and lumpy at the beginning and white or yellowish in color, improves greatly in the following days. Large amounts of water are brought along and added, causing the mucus to become more transparent and much more watery. More and more mucus trickles out of the cervix and flows down through the vagina, where you may feel and see it.

Entrance to the Cervix: The Gate of Life Opens

The Estrogen Friends ensure that the Gate of Life (the cervix) opens, and boost the blood circulation so that it feels much softer and smoother. The support ligaments of the uterus become tighter, and in some cases the cervix moves upwards.

> **FACT**
> *The luteinizing hormone can only be released from the pituitary gland when the estrogens have been at a highly concentrated level in the blood for a certain length of time. This causes ovulation to take place about 9 to 24 hours later.*

Control Center: The Ovulation Helpers Prepare for Action

The Estrogen Friends are also transported via the bloodstream to the brain. At the beginning there are only very few of them, but as the egg ripens more and more estrogens arrive on the scene. The estrogens job here is to constantly repeat the same request for help: "Down in the ovary, the egg will soon be mature and is preparing for her adventurous journey. It won't be long now and she'll need your help, she can't manage this leap by herself." A special team is sent from the pituitary gland in the "Control Center" for this big event. These are the "Ovulation Helpers", also referred to as the luteinizing hormone (LH).

Ovulation: The Adventurous Leap

Meanwhile, in the ovary, the follicle has reached maturity and has a diameter of about .8 inches (2cm), and the Queen Egg inside is now fully grown and prepared for the adventure ahead. The fallopian tube, normally not connected to the ovary, starts to move. It comes closer and closer, and with its finger-shaped end places itself on the spot where the follicle bulges out from the ovary.

When the cover bursts, the egg will be gently caught and slipped into the funnel shaped opening so that it won't fall deep into the abdomen and get lost forever. The egg has just a few hours of life left now.

The Ovulation Helpers (LH) dash off from the pituitary gland in the direction of the ovary, and with their help the follicle's protective cover splits open in the hours that follow. The liquid is projected out of the follicle, and if all goes well, the precious egg is safely caught by the fallopian tube. It doesn't know yet what lies ahead; will it meet with a sperm or will its life soon be over?

FACT
According to recent studies, the estrogens are also responsible for gentle muscle contractions of the uterus, resulting in a kind of suction at the cervix. This results in groups of sperm being moved upwards as if using a lift. On the side of the ovary with the Queen Egg, there is a higher concentration of estrogens than on the other side. Via a small direct bloodstream, this high estrogen level reaches the tiny muscles of the uterine end of the fallopian tube, causing the sperm to be sucked into the tube.

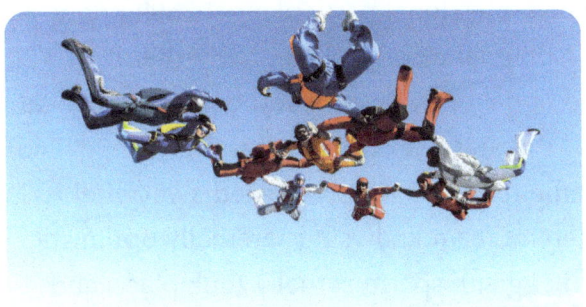

The luteinising hormone (LH) is sent by the pituitary gland down to the ovary where it causes ovulation to occur.

The Estrogen Friends have done their job for the time being; they withdraw from the different places of action (uterus, cervical mucus glands etc.) and take a well-earned break. The protective cover of the follicle is now empty and left behind in the ovary, where it collapses and sometimes bleeds a little. You might think that things will finally quiet down here, after all, the egg is gone, therefore the work must surely be over, right? The first act of the Cycle Show may have come to an end; however the ovary will once again be the scene where lots of new happenings take place during the second act.

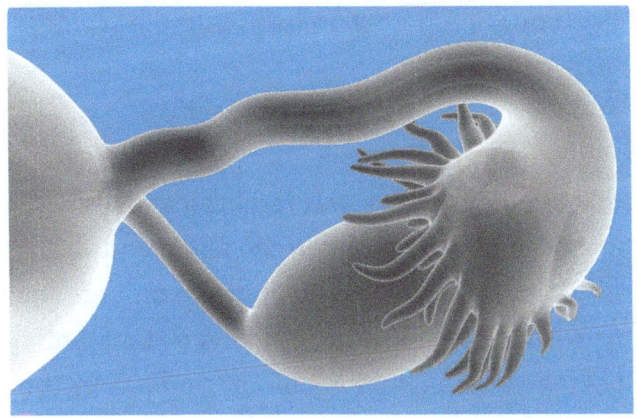

Before ovulation the fingers of the fallopian tube place themselves over the ovary, exactly above the mature follicle, in order to carefully catch the egg when it bursts out.

Second Act of the Cycle Show – The Service Center Goes into Action

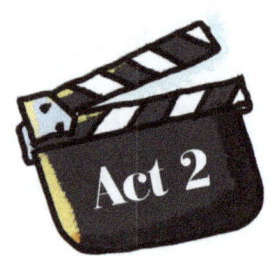

We now bring color onto the stage. The empty follicle changes into a yellow body called the corpus luteum, named because doctors noticed it took on this yellow color after ovulation. A little unimaginative maybe, but back then they didn't really know exactly what they were dealing with. Nowadays it would probably be called the "Service Center."

So who works here at the Service Center? A few of the Estrogen Friends are still here in the second act of the Cycle Show. They continue to look after the woman's well-being in the background, but the scene is now clearly dominated by the progesterone.

The "Progesterone Team" is a highly skilled group of professional party planners, who now very carefully prepare the woman's body for a possible pregnancy regardless of whether it happens or not. As you know, following ovulation the signal between egg and body was lost, so the newly fledged Progesterone Team doesn't know at this stage what happened to the egg. Did the egg meet a sperm or remain alone? Or did it become tired and simply wasted away after its very short lifespan? Anyone familiar with the Progesterone Team knows it is eternally optimistic, therefore it assumes that the great encounter between egg and sperm actually took place, and that a new life is now on its way to the womb.

Uterine Hotel: Interior Decoration of the Luxury Suites

Imagine that the egg was fertilized and a small guest can now be found in the fallopian tube. It makes its way towards the uterus in order to look for a cozy place to settle. But how is it currently looking in there at the moment? So far only the foundations are ready; it's really still a building site! The rooms on the top floor of the hotel are completely bare and not very inviting. There's a lot of work waiting for the Progesterone Team. Upon their instruction, lots of tiny blood vessels sprout in the top layer of the uterine lining, glands develop, and vital nutrients (sugar, proteins, vitamins, antibodies, and minerals)

> **FACT**
> The first phase of the cycle has many names: the follicular phase, the egg ripening phase, the estrogen phase or the proliferation phase. It lasts from the first day of menstruation until ovulation.

are stored everywhere. The Progesterone Team continues to work tirelessly to decorate and furnish the hotel with cushions and blankets. About a week after ovulation, in the middle of the second phase of the cycle, everything is ready. A small guest could now look for a place to nestle down and make itself comfortable, in the luxuriously furnished uterine lining.

End of Season: No more Magic Potion
Shortly before ovulation the Estrogen Friends had finished their task in the Leisure Center and had departed. When the Progesterone Team arrive, the season is completely over. The glands are shut down, and they make sure that the Magic Potion is no longer available. The previous day's cervical mucus was possibly still clear and runny, but it has now come to an end overnight. From now on a thick mucus plug seals the entrance to the uterus, even tighter and more impenetrable than at the beginning of the cycle.

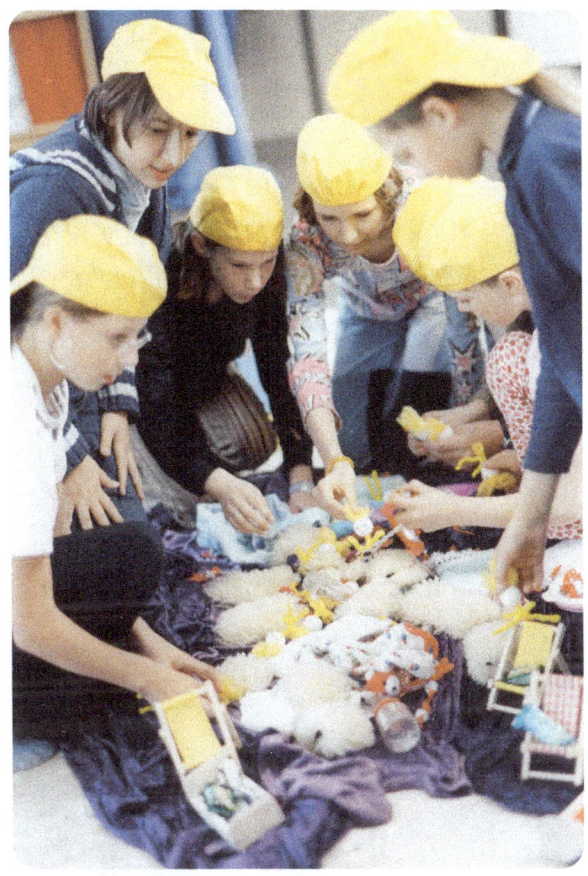

The Progesterone Team have about a week after ovulation to furnish the uterine lining with everything a baby could need.

The Gate of Life is Locked
The opening of the cervix becomes smaller again and the Gate of Life is firmly locked. What's going on here is completely understandable, as it would be pointless for more sperm to enter as they wouldn't meet an egg. Bacteria should not be allowed to enter in order to protect the woman, and also a baby, if it is growing inside her. If a baby is in there, the cervix has to be closed so the baby stays inside the uterus until it's time to be born.

Preparation of Mammary Glands: Milk for the Baby
The activities started by the Progesterone Team are now almost bordering on over eagerness. The baby needs milk from the mother's breast soon after it is born, therefore everything should be prepared so the infant can be fed immediately. Why the big rush so early on? Although it's not yet clear if there will be any need for it, the first preparations for the milk production are always started in the second act of the Cycle Show. Right after ovulation, when the corpus luteum sends off the

Progesterone Team, the blood supply to the breasts is raised and additional mammary glands start growing. It's a time consuming process, one which is nine months long.

Temperature Rises: The Progesterone Team Warm Things up

In addition to preparing the mammary glands, another remarkable change takes place. We're talking about our own central heating system, which makes sure that our bodies are kept at the right temperature. Like all important control centers, this is found in the brain and is known as the temperature regulating center.

A woman's body temperature is somewhat lower in the first phase of the cycle. The Progesterone Team is responsible for raising the body's temperature of 98.6°F by about one degree around the time of ovulation, when the corpus luteum starts to work. The temperature remains at this higher level until the end of the cycle or, if a pregnancy has occurred, for the next months.

> **FACT**
> The second phase of the cycle also has many names: the luteal phase, progesterone phase, or the secretion phase. This lasts from ovulation until the day before the period.

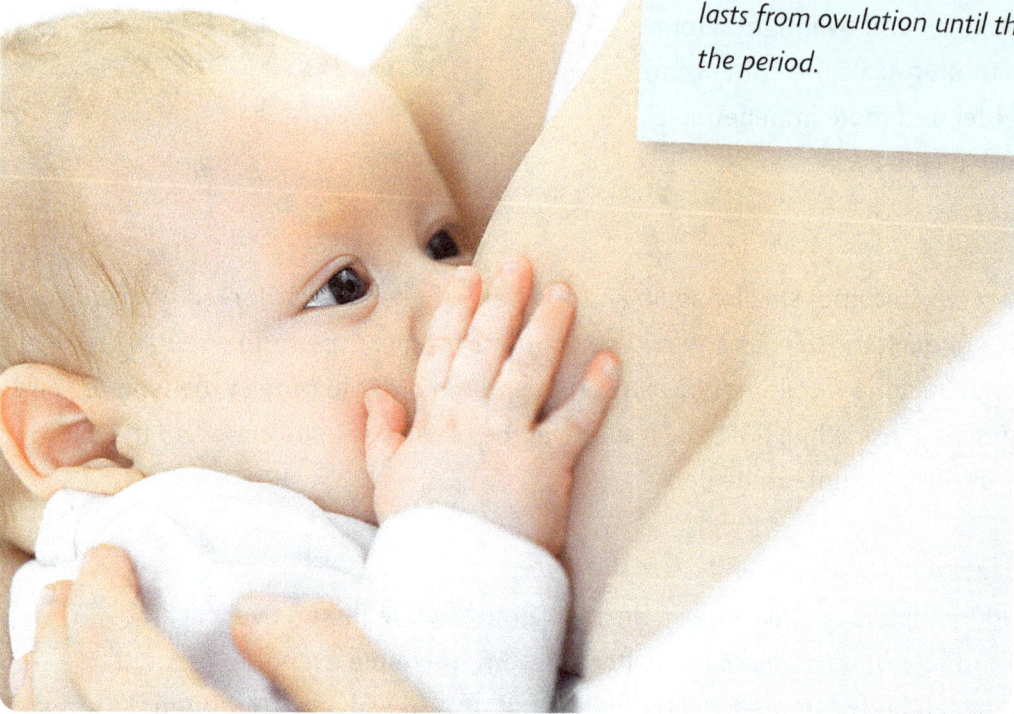

The mammary glands are prepared for possible milk production by the Progesterone Team in every second phase of the cycle.

The Shutdown Agreement Applies to the Managers in the Control Center

The final task for the Progesterone Team is to let the managers in the Control Center know that preparations for a possible pregnancy are running at full steam. It goes without saying that the managers should not disturb these activities. A "Shutdown Agreement" is put into place. This is a very strict law stating that as long as the corpus luteum is doing its work and the Progesterone Team is preparing all the organs in the body for a pregnancy, then all activities should come to a standstill in the ovary.

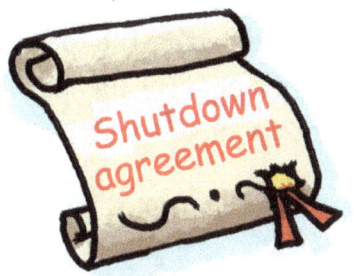

> **FACT**
> The biological term for the Shutdown Agreement is the "negative feedback mechanism of the hormonal cycle." This is a complex physiological mechanism which ensures that following a possible fertilization, a second opportunity to fertilize an egg will not occur.

Therefore:
- No Messengers of Spring are allowed to be sent out
- No further eggs are allowed to mature

During this time, no other ovulation may take place until it is clear whether or not the egg and sperm have found each other.

Absolutely Infertile

Following ovulation in the second act of the Cycle Show, when the Progesterone Team is active:
- The cervix is tightly closed.
- The sperm cannot survive without the Magic Potion.
- Due to the Shutdown Agreement, no further eggs are allowed to mature and thus no ovulation occurs.

Therefore in the second phase of the cycle a woman cannot get pregnant anymore.

As a consequence, this phase after ovulation is called the "absolutely infertile" phase of the cycle.

Grand Finale and Small Finale

So how does the story end? There are two different final scenes; a grand and a small finale.

The "Grand Finale" occurs less often nowadays, although everything points to it having been the original script for the end of the show. When egg and sperm meet and merge together, new life begins. The embryo settles down happily in the uterine hotel, restoring contact with its mother and sending her its very first love letter. Nine months later, now fully grown, the baby is born and finally sees the light of day. That's the Grand Finale of the Cycle Show.

More commonly however, the situation in a woman's body is completely different. The sperm doesn't even appear on the scene in the Cycle Show and is unable to meet the egg. The uterine hotel remains empty, and no hormone (HGC) will inform the woman's body about a baby's arrival.

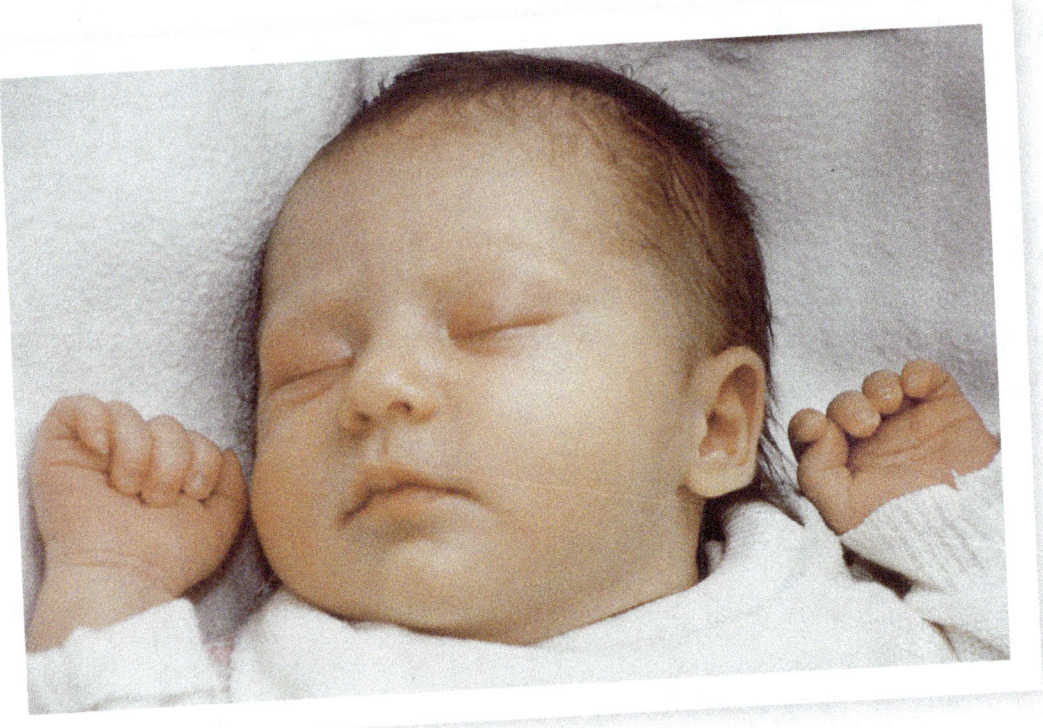

The Birth of a Child – The Grand Finale of the Cycle Show.

Everyone would have been waiting for this message, especially the corpus luteum which spent the whole week preparing everything so professionally. Now the mailbox remains empty; there's no love letter, text message, or even an e-mail arriving this time. Eventually it becomes clear to the corpus luteum: "Okay. Nothing happened in this cycle, perhaps next time around."

An Honorable Retreat: Making Way for a New Opportunity

Within the next few days the corpus luteum calls the Progesterone Team back from the places where they have been so busy. The party planners did an excellent job, but they won't be needed any more. The corpus luteum, the key player of this second phase of the cycle, stops its hormone production about 10 to 16 days after ovulation and leaves the stage.

There are consequences in the uterus as well. Although the Progesterone Team would have liked to stay here for a while longer, they realize that the quicker they leave the stage now, the sooner they'll get another chance. As a Grand Finale is what they are longing for, they take their leave and retreat from the uterine hotel in order to try again.

What happens now with all the luxurious items? They can't be left behind as the body is an exclusive five-star hotel. When something is specially prepared for one guest, it can't be served up again for another. Each guest gets the best service, everything freshly and individually prepared. When the completely fresh and richly furnished suite (the top layer of the uterine lining) is no longer needed, it flows out of the body with the blood. This is the "Small Finale" of the Cycle Show, known as the monthly period.

> **FACT**
> Visualize the blood as a means of transport, in which all nutrients that are no longer needed for a guest, flow out of our body.

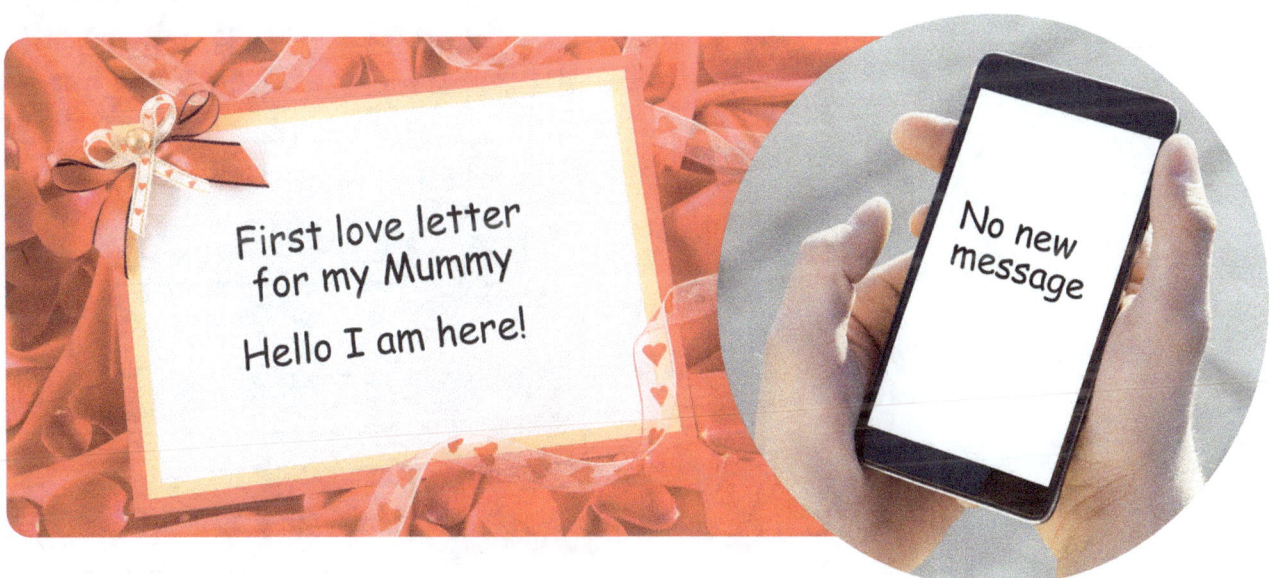

If the corpus luteum has waited in vain for a message, then it withdraws the Progesterone Team from the body – the Small Finale takes place!

The Cycle Show

1. Control Center (brain) sends the Messengers of Spring (FSH) to the ovary.
2. Eggs are woken up, follicles develop and estrogens are produced.
3. Estrogens construct the uterine lining.
4. Estrogens open the season at the cervical glands: Magic Potion is produced.
5. In the days before and around ovulation, sperm can survive well in the cervical mucus – good times for the sperm!
6. Control Center sends Ovulation Helpers (LH) to the ovary.
7. Ovulation
8. Corpus luteum is active and produces progesterone.
9. Shutdown Agreement is made between the brain and the progesterone.
10. Progesterone decorates and furnishes the luxurious uterine lining.
11. Progesterone stops the season at the cervical mucus glands.
12. Progesterone causes the body temperature to rise about one degree F
13. In the second phase of the cycle, the cervix is sealed tightly—bad times for the sperm!

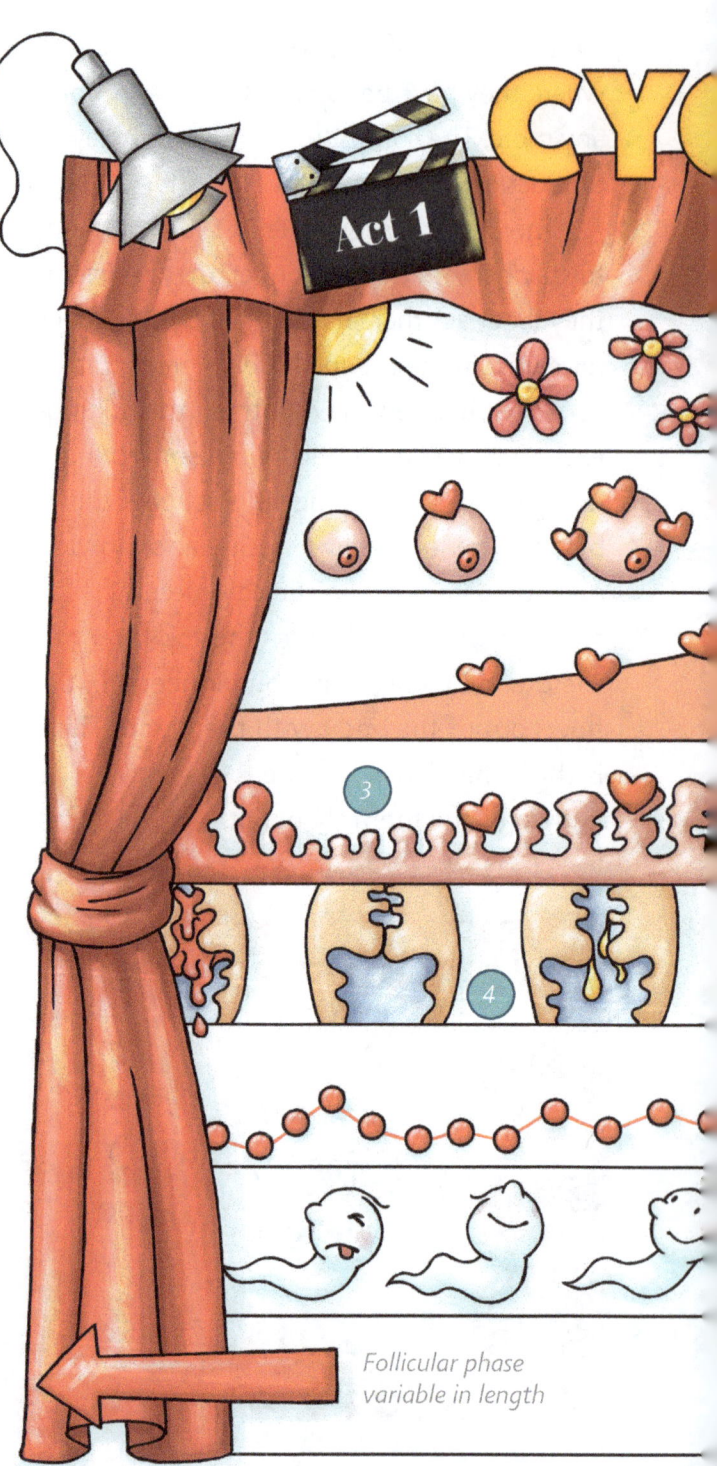

Follicular phase variable in length

The Cycle Show

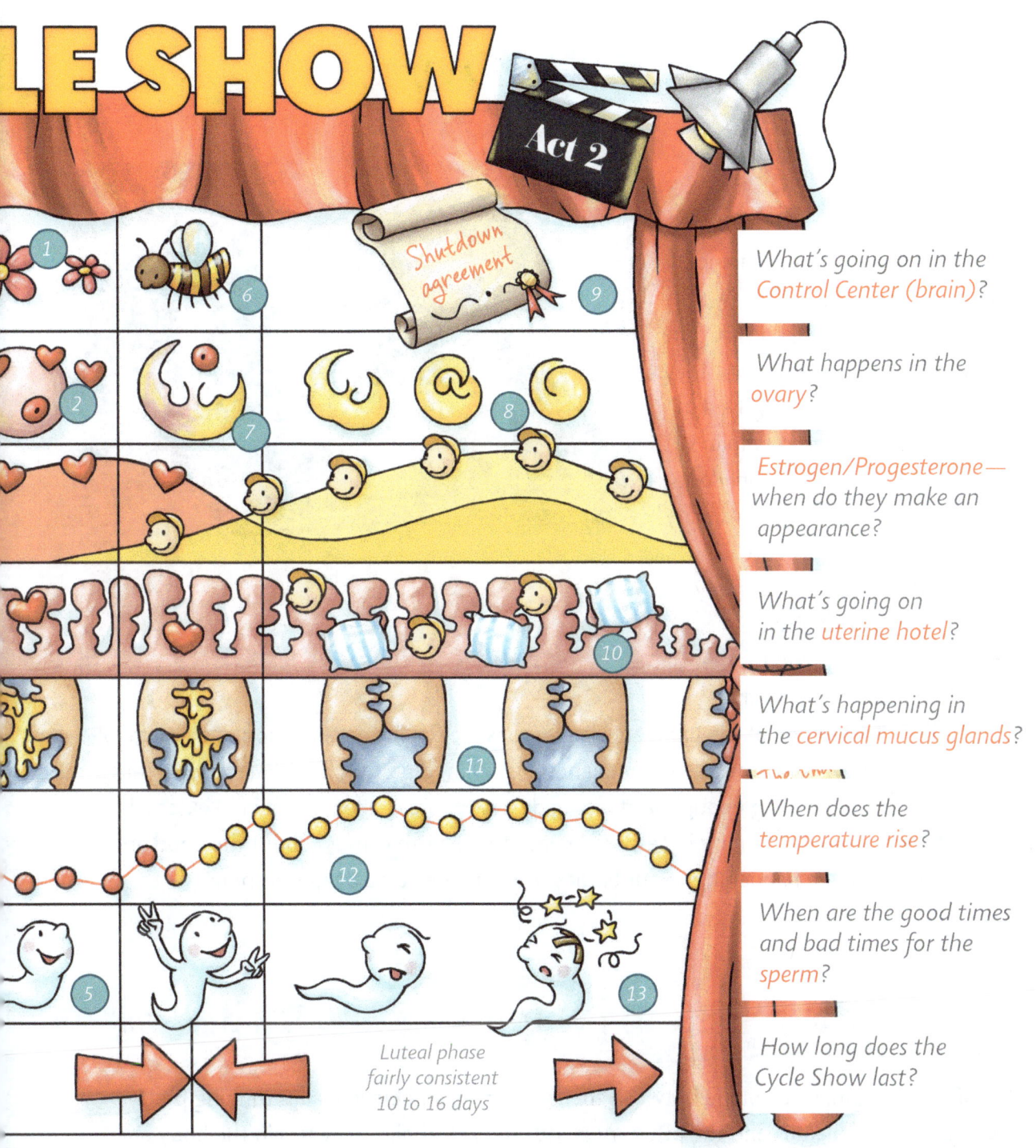

Act 2

What's going on in the Control Center (brain)?

What happens in the ovary?

Estrogen/Progesterone— when do they make an appearance?

What's going on in the uterine hotel?

What's happening in the cervical mucus glands?

When does the temperature rise?

When are the good times and bad times for the sperm?

How long does the Cycle Show last?

Luteal phase fairly consistent 10 to 16 days

5 Puberty and the Premiere of the Cycle Show

Senior Management in the Control Center

In the previous chapter the appearance of the managers in our brain (the hypothalamus and the pituitary gland) in our Cycle Show was definitely too short, they are undoubtedly much more involved in the success of the whole process than we can imagine. The Cycle Show is only one among many other areas of responsibility for the senior management in the brain. The hypothalamus and pituitary gland are in charge of our physical and mental development, and for the regulation of our breathing and the

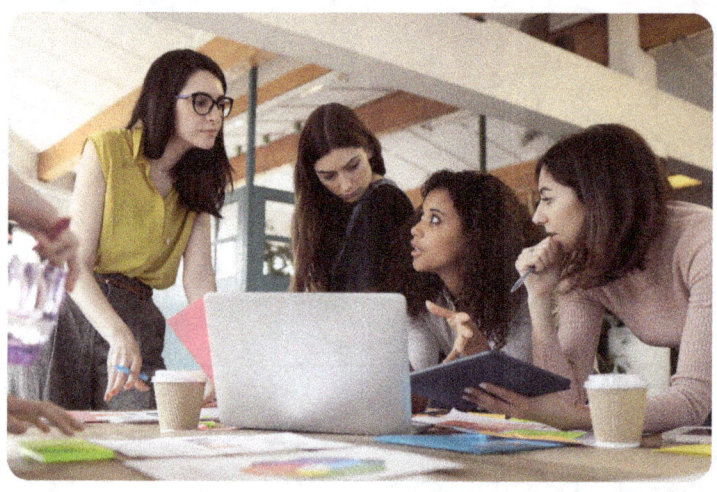

The hypothalamus and pituitary gland make up the Control Center in charge of the numerous processes in our body. Both negative and positive stimuli from the environment can influence them.

circulatory system. These parts of the brain are also responsible for the organization of all metabolic processes, for the kidneys, sodium and water balance, nutrition, digestion, and much more. These daily routine jobs are demanding enough, but are made even more challenging by the external messages that are continually pouring in (especially into the hypothalamus) about the good and not so good things that are happening in our bodies. There needs to be a rapid response to these messages.

The Cycle Show Section is Open – Puberty Begins

In the life of a young girl, somewhere between the age of nine and eleven, all is running pretty smoothly in the hypothalamus and the pituitary gland. The metabolic processes in the body are working well, and the body weight and growth are healthy for her age. Everything is just fine!

When a stable state has been reached, one can afford to focus on the beautiful things in life and give little thought to the future. When you are tall, mature and strong enough, the managers in the brain decide it's time for puberty to start. The managers in charge of the Cycle Show begin their work by sending the Messengers of Spring (follicle stimulating hormone) to both ovaries for the very first time, where about 400,000 eggs have been hibernating since birth. When this hormone arrives at the ovaries, it gently coaxes a few of the eggs to come to life. It takes a little while to convince the sleepy heads to wake up and go into action, but sooner or later they become aware of the excitement that lies ahead.

Estrogens Transform a Girl into a Woman

The Start of a Long Friendship
The initial follicles now begin to grow and the first Estrogen Friends develop on the protective cover. Shortly afterwards, they spread out for the first time all over your body, and with a lot of flair and imagination, they transform you from a girl into a woman.

It Starts with a Small Pearl: Breast Development
Around the same time as the onset of the first pubic hair, the Estrogen Friends start the breast development. To begin with it feels like there's a small pearl under each nipple which gets a little bigger every day.
Then finally it's more like a soft, round cushion which can really hurt if you accidentally bump it into something.

FACT
At puberty, there are not only female hormones being produced, but also the male hormone testosterone. Testosterone is responsible for activating the sweat, sebaceous, and scent glands, which you can identify by the fact that your hair gets greasier, you may get acne, and you need to shower more often. Pubic and underarm hair grow under the influence of this male hormone.

FACT
Nature planned for the pubic hair at the entrance of the vagina to be additional protection for the precious Stage of Life, preventing larger particles from entering.

The best baby food in the world is made in the breasts, which are also called mammary glands. These glands will be built at the very beginning of puberty by our Estrogen Friends. We could compare the mammary glands with a very delicate and valuable china tea cup, which should be wrapped extremely carefully so it can't be damaged. The wrapping, which is made of fat tissue, is missing in the beginning because the glands develop first. This is the reason why our glands are painful if you touch them accidentally, until they are protected with fat tissue they can really hurt. The fat, or adipose tissue, differs quite a lot from woman to woman. If a woman has a lot of adipose tissue then a woman will have large breasts, if another woman has less than she will have smaller breasts. It's all quite normal as the Estrogen Friends like to put great emphasis on individuality.

    The Estrogen Friends cause your breasts to grow. It is possible that initially one breast grows faster than the other, as more estrogens go to one side before going to the other. But don't worry, it will catch up later and you won't see a difference. Just remind yourself that this is typical of best friends, they always want to do things together! Gradually the nipples and the surrounding area, called the areola, also become larger and darker. Breast development is usually not complete until about 17 years of age.

Just like Artists, Estrogen Friends Form your Body

At puberty your body shape changes and becomes typically feminine; your waist gets narrower, the hips wider, and the bottom a little rounder. The labia become larger and grow to varying sizes, and sometimes the inner labia are bigger than the outer ones. This is also quite normal. The skin in the vulval area, the area between your legs, becomes darker and the uterus and the vagina both grow too. You'll experience a growth spurt, usually starting shortly after the breast development begins,

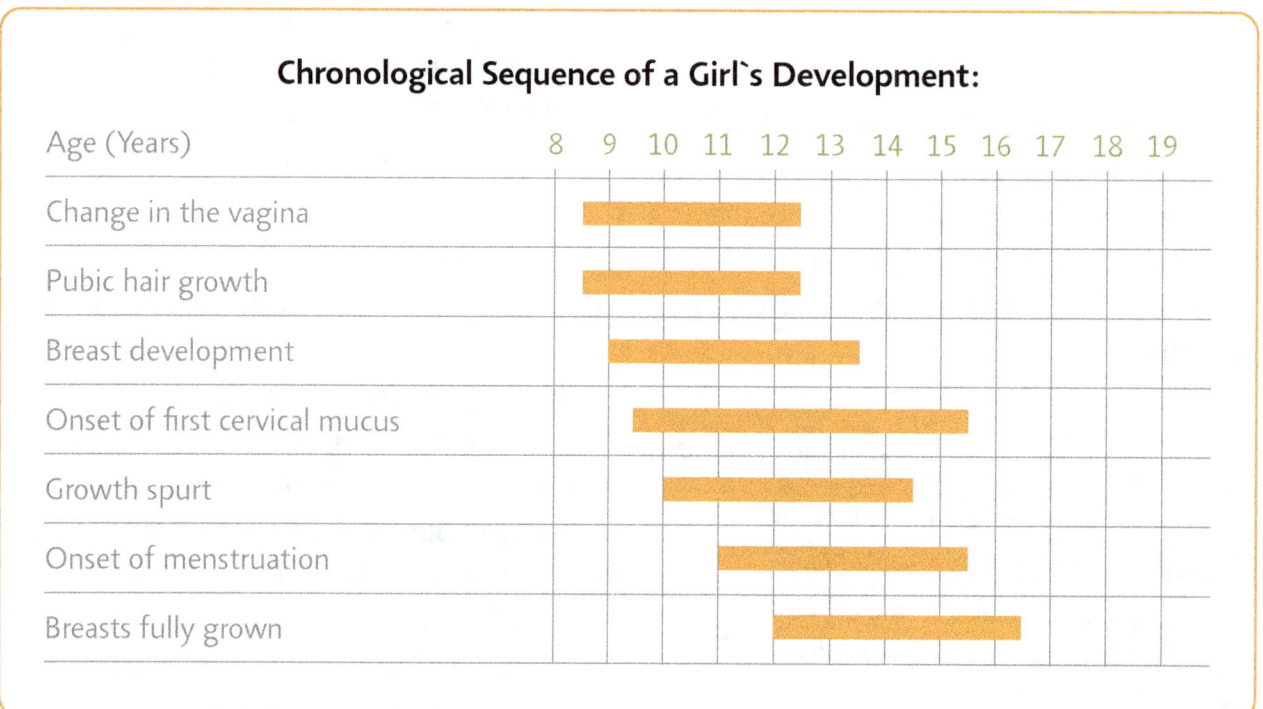

growing around 4-8 inches in height and putting on 4-5 pounds in weight. A certain minimum weight is necessary in order for menstruation to begin, which is why low body weight can be a reason for the first period not starting.

The Estrogen Friends are artists who take great care with their work and the task of changing you into a woman. The estrogens will look after you for many years, just like best friends do. They'll keep your bones strong and healthy, protect your blood vessels from dangerous deposits, make your hair shiny, your nails strong, your skin smell good, and your mucus membranes moist and healthy. Your Estrogen Friends will even give you your very own unique, distinctive look.

Not a Child Anymore but not yet a Woman! The Rollercoaster of Emotions

You may already know this situation, or you will soon. During the years when the Cycle Show is still being rehearsed in your body, everything feels topsy-turvy in your life and nothing is the way it used to be. It's not just your body that's changing; your heart and soul discover a whole new world also. It's a huge change when the Estrogen Friends suddenly arrive in the brain and start to interfere with your moods and feelings, turning everything upside down. For the first time you will begin to experience a longing for affection. The Estrogen Friends will wake up your desire and the wonderful feelings of being in love, and they will also be responsible for the fact that at other times you may feel sad. At these times you may feel down in the dumps, and life may not feel easy. This time of change can feel difficult to you, but be patient and kind to yourself and trust that all will be well. When the Estrogen Friends become part of your life, you won't feel or see things like a child anymore, but like a woman. They will accompany you over many years, helping you to feel comfortable in your more womanly body.

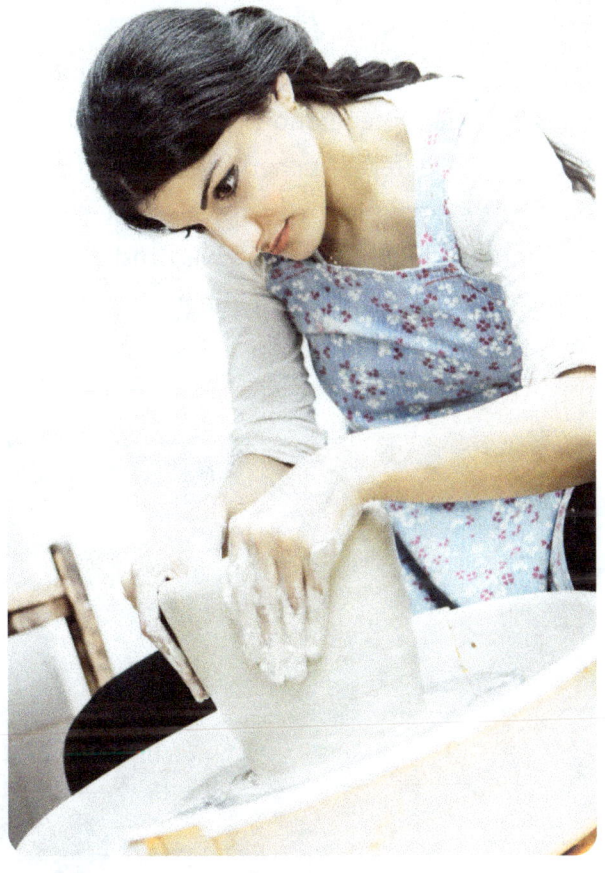

The Estrogen Friends are like artists who go to work long before the first period, changing the body of a girl into that of a young woman.

Changes on the Stage of Life

The First Foundations are Laid in the Uterine Hotel

So, what happens next? Do the Estrogen Friends start to set up the uterine lining at this early stage of puberty and begin preparing the foundations for the Luxury Suites? Although it is still early and they could wait a couple of years, they actually do head there. As soon as the first estrogens swarm all over the body through the bloodstream, they start to build up the uterine lining. Everything is new and unfamiliar as they have had no practice, which is why they naturally take longer the first time. Initially, the preparation of your body and your uterine hotel for the Special Guest that might arrive can last months, or even two to three years, from the beginning of puberty until the first period. Later on, as an experienced team, it will only take two to three weeks to complete this task.

The Leisure Center (Spa) is Open

Of course the estrogens also go to the cervix during the first preparations. This means that the Leisure Center is opened for the very first time. The mucus plug, which sealed the cervix throughout childhood, is removed and the cervical mucus glands slowly begin to prepare the first Magic Potion under the direction of the estrogens.

> **FACT**
> Many women have little understanding about the real meaning of their cervical mucus. This became clear in a survey of 5500 girls in a medical clinic in Vienna, where one in three girls came to the clinic with a cervical mucus discharge, believing they were ill.

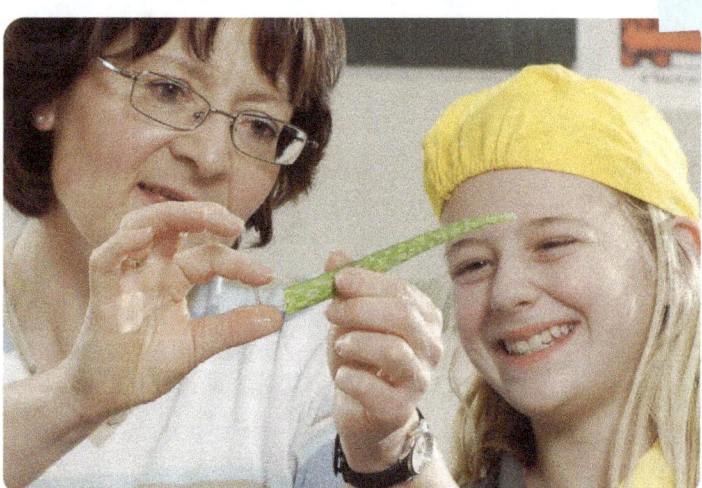

The cervical mucus resembles the appearance of the liquid of the Aloe Vera plant.

Many girls who don't know the secret code of their bodies may start to get worried. One day they notice a strange whitish or yellowish mucus in their underwear or notice when they wipe themselves after going to the bathroom, the paper slides over the vaginal entrance as if oiled. They see a whitish or sometimes clear, slippery mucus, sort of like raw egg white on the toilet paper. If a girl doesn't know what that means, it can make her feel rather worried.

Puberty and the Premiere of the Cycle Show

Some girls are brave and ask their mother, female friend or older sister what the mucus is. Often they hear that this is "normal" in puberty and some are told more precisely that it's the first mucus that all girls have before their first period. Sometimes worried mothers take their daughters to the doctor when this occurs for the first time, as they're afraid that this "discharge" may be an infection. You will never have these worries as you know that long before your first period, when you notice lumpy, whitish mucus:

> *There's no need for a hygiene drama because of the appearance of the first mucus! It's a sign that you are healthy. Just wash yourself as usual and change your underwear daily.*

- The managers in my Control Center have started the Cycle Show.
- The first eggs are ripening in my ovaries.
- My best friends, the estrogens, are already at work, looking after me and changing me from a girl into a woman.
- My uterine lining will be created for the first time.
- Cervical mucus, which is vitally important for the creation of a new life, is also being produced for the first time at the cervix. Without this cervical mucus, I wouldn't even exist.
- I'm not ill; in fact my body is healthy and working well!

After the first sign of mucus it can take up to two years before the first period comes. With time it appears more frequently, becoming clearer, more liquid and stretchy, like raw egg white. When the vaginal area feels moist you know that soon you will get your first period and experience the first Small Finale of the Cycle Show!

AMY (12)

Last week I went to the doctor for the first time. I'd been having a strange whitish discharge, so for weeks my mother has tried to encourage me to see the doctor. First I really didn't want to go, I found it totally embarrassing. In the end I agreed and was lucky, it was a very nice lady doctor who simply asked me some questions. She gave me a detailed explanation about the cervical mucus. As the mucus is not itchy, doesn't burn or have an unpleasant smell and since it comes and goes, she was sure it is my cervical mucus.

The Premiere: The First Period, the Menarche

Sooner or later your first period will happen. A few weeks before your first period, a Queen Egg will be selected for the first time. After a time of maturation, she will be ready for her big adventure: the first ovulation. This great event will happen about two weeks before your first menstruation. After this the first corpus luteum will develop, and the Progesterone Team will start with the luxurious preparations of the uterine lining. For the first time, the task of clearing up will lie ahead. This will be the premiere, the first Small Finale.

> **FACT**
> Only 2% of girls start their menarche (first period) at the age of 10. At the age of 14, about 90% of the girls have had their first period.

> **FACT**
> Ovulation doesn't always occur before the first period. It is possible that only the "foundations," built up by the estrogens over several months, bleed out of the uterus. The blood itself is not a clear indication whether ovulation took place or not.

Worthy of a Bunch of Flowers: Entering Womanhood

For the very first time, your body gives you the strongest signal it possibly can that it has made the transition from being a girl to a woman; you now have the ability to bring new life into the world.

The first period, called menarche, is a unique moment in your life. When you hear women talking about it, it's clear that for most of them this is a day they remember, alongside the day they gave birth to their children. It goes without saying that this premiere needs to be celebrated!

It's fully understandable if you don't feel like celebrating; maybe you have been surprised by your first period and are unsure how you feel about it.

You know that the first period is something private which sadly is not discussed openly in our society. Even if you are delighted, you may

> **FACT**
> Can a girl become pregnant before her first period? Theoretically, yes! Roughly two weeks before the first period the first egg could possibly be in the fallopian tube where it could be fertilized.

> **FACT**
> There is a rare, hereditary blood clotting disorder called von Willebrand disease. Often it emerges when girls have their first period. When the first bleed is extremely heavy, and continues for a long time, one should consider this - especially if the mother usually has very long and heavy periods.

find it embarrassing to talk about and afraid of someone making a silly comment. Don't be discouraged! Don't let this day go by like any other. Look for a circle of people you trust (mother, aunt, big sister, or friend) and celebrate your birth into womanhood with them, possibly doing something special.

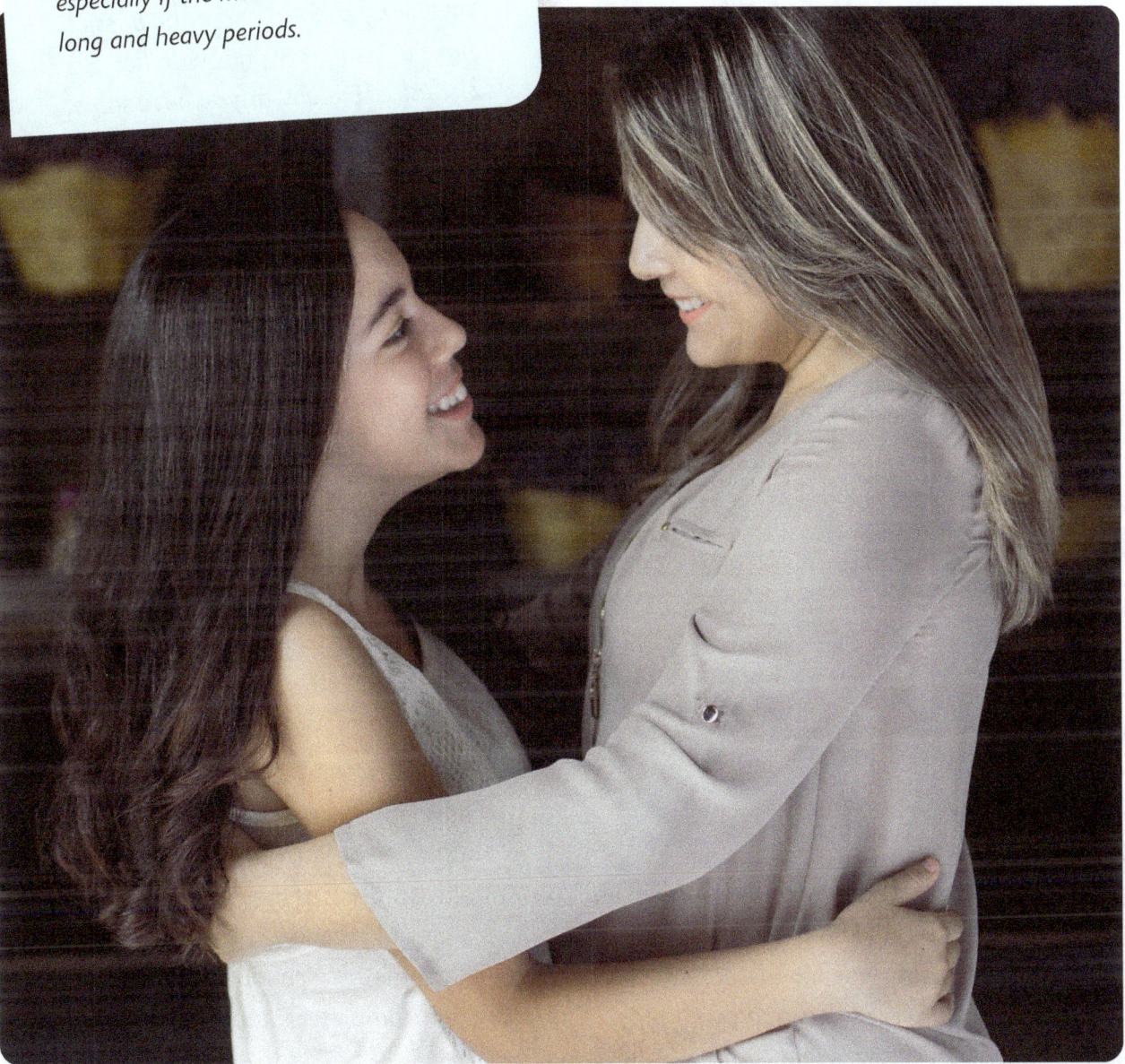

The first period, called menarche, is a unique moment in your life and needs to be celebrated!

Puberty and the Premiere of the Cycle Show

No Panic: When the Time Comes, You'll Have a Good Understanding Now

A lot of girls are afraid that their first period will take them by surprise at a really inconvenient moment; at the swimming pool, in a restaurant or on a vacation. They imagine losing lots of

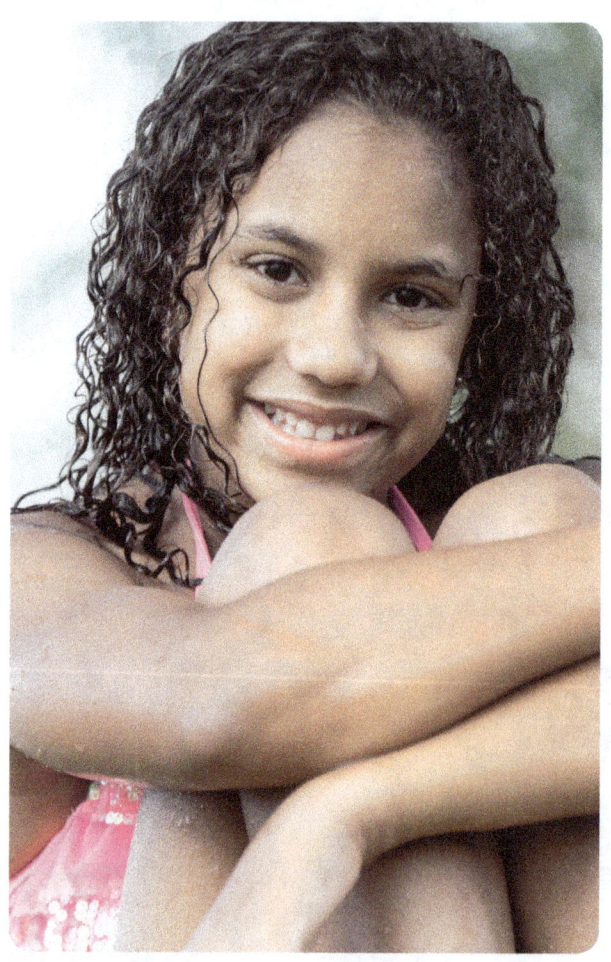

> A class of girls had a lesson telling them the real meaning of their periods. Shortly afterwards they came to a decision: "As of today, if one of us starts her period she declares it to the class by saying "listen girls, I got my luxury today!" and if she doesn't have any sanitary pads with her she asks: "Do any of you have some luxury articles with you?"

blood and everyone being able to see it. But don't worry! For most girls the period begins with very light bleeding, which often looks like a brownish shimmer on the toilet paper. If you have no sanitary pad on hand it's not the end of the world, paper tissues or toilet paper will do. It is very rare for a lot of blood to flow out of the vagina at the very beginning, but even if this were to happen don't let it worry you. Confide in a friend or an older woman you trust, she'll be very kind and understanding. If your pants have got some blood on them then you can tie your sweatshirt around your hips and remind yourself that what comes out of your body is "pure luxury."

BECKY (14)

When I started my period, we didn't have any sanitary pads or tampons at home, because my mother had already reached menopause. She was all flustered and ran around looking for something suitable for me to use. I felt completely stupid.

EMMA (18)

I didn't start my periods until I was 16. We had been to the doctor before that but he said that everything was quite normal. I longed to be just like all the other girls my age! It was such a relief when I had my first period. I was delighted! I am still always glad when it starts, because I am still fairly irregular. I can't imagine ever seeing my period as a nuisance, even if I sometimes have a stomach ache. I view it as a sign of being a woman in good health.

STEPH (17)

I was only nine when I had my first period. My mom told me later that she had never spoken about it "because I was so young." I think that was a mistake, but maybe I wouldn't have understood much of what was ahead of me. When it began, it was dreadful. I wished that it would stop again, and it actually stayed away for a year. It's only now that I've come to terms with my cycle. I read a few good books by women, for women. That helped.

JESS (13)

My mother suggested a couple of months before my first period that we should go shopping to buy sanitary pads. I could not see the point, as there were always some lying around in the bathroom cabinet. She probably just wanted an excuse to bring up the subject. I already knew all about it from my friend, who had started her periods much earlier. When the time came, it was quite normal for me. It was no big deal. The following weekend my parents took me out to a fancy restaurant "in honor of the occasion."

LILLY (15)

I was away for a few days visiting my aunt when my period started. Of course, I had nothing with me. I was embarrassed to say anything, so at first I stuffed toilet paper and paper tissues into my pants. (I often still do that when it takes me by surprise). By the evening, I had to tell my aunt, because she had noticed I was behaving strangely. She was so kind to me and the next morning there was a bunch of flowers in front of my breakfast plate and everyone acted as if it were my birthday.

Historical Premiere Celebrations from all over the World

It is said that in many **Indian cultures of North and South America**, the menarche celebration was the most important religious-social event. A little while before the celebration, in a hut of her own, the girl was let in on the female secrets by an experienced woman. Following a short fasting period, she would be led to a tribal celebration given in her honor, which lasted for several days. She was festively dressed and painted, and performed a ritual dance which established her new status as a woman.

In **Panama** it is said that the Kuna Indian tribe celebrates an Inna-Festival in honor of all girls who have just had their menarche. As a sign of their female dignity a red scarf, richly decorated with gold embroidery, is tied around their head. They wear bright red and gold shirts as a symbol of fertility. The fathers gather leaves from sacred trees for the ceremonial rituals.

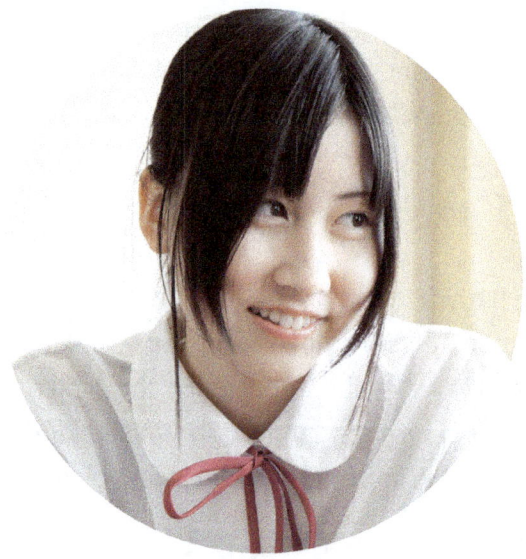

People say that in **Japan** the young girls' "first blossom festival" is celebrated. When the guests arrive to the festive dinner, they come to understand the reason for the celebration because of the red blossoms and candied apples with which the table is decorated. On some Japanese islands it is said that the menarche celebration has an even greater importance than a wedding.

It is said that in one tribe in **Colorado** the father makes a proud announcement to the whole tribe that his daughter is to be consecrated a woman. During a smoke ceremony a wise woman scatters fragrant grasses, cedar needles and sage on a piece of coal. The girl bows over the smoke, and in so doing asks the protective spirits of nature to give her health and fertility.

It is understood that in a tribe in **Brazil** the girl gets a new haircut upon her first menstruation. The childish braids are cut off, and a pretty fringe hairstyle shows that the girl has turned into a young woman. Relatives and friends receive a wisp of hair as a keepsake.

In some regions of **Nigeria** it is said that when a girl has her first period she is seen as a person who contributes to fertility and thus brings good luck. On this day she walks through all the village fields, letting a few drops of her blood flow onto the soil which blesses the land to bring a rich harvest.

Aboriginal Australians celebrated the menarche with a big party, rejoicing the female power which was now at home in a young girl with dance and song.

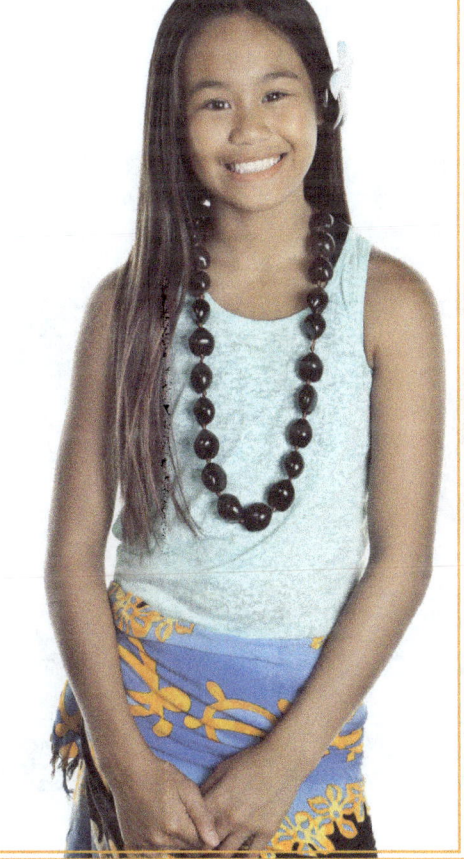

6 The Small Finale–My Period

Menstrual bleeding is the most impressive sign given by the body during the Cycle Show. It accompanies every woman, month after month, for about 400 cycles over a time span of 35 to 40 years.

It is quite surprising that this event is discussed so infrequently, and if it should come up, then it's often about hygienic measures, discomfort, and problems. Science has even gone as far as trying to rid women of this "bothersome nuisance" altogether. If women are only informed about the "renovation work" in their bodies and not about everything else that is taking place, then they are lacking in information. Taken out of its natural context, the period can be an inconvenience and may appear unnecessary, but when women know about the Cycle Show in their body, then they are able to understand what this period really means. It is both the end and the beginning of a wonderful drama, a sign of luxury, richness, and abundance. The period really is worth talking about!

> **FACT**
> There are many different expressions for the period: menstruation, bleeding, period, and time of the month.

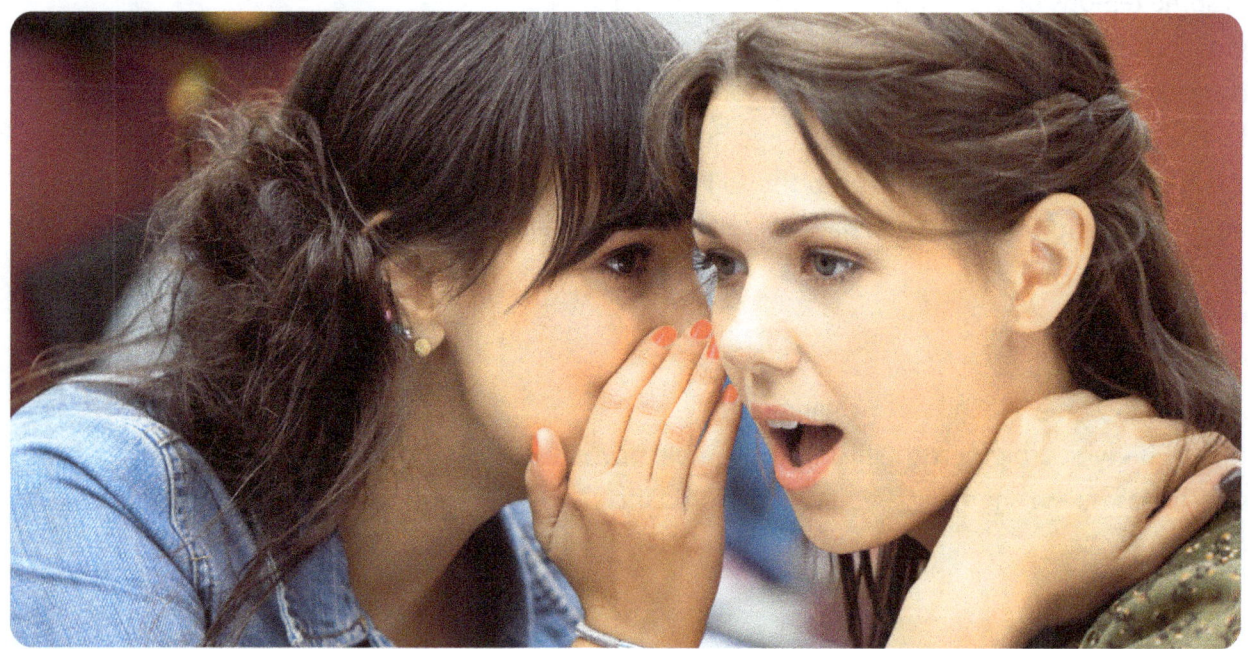

"My period" – a subject which is still not openly discussed.

Blood is the Essence of Life

What do you feel when you see blood? Fear maybe, or horror and disgust? Some people may say they can't stand the sight of it. Nobody is indifferent to blood; it awakens unpleasant feelings that are connected to sickness and the fear of death. When blood is flowing, then normally something dreadful has happened: an accident, injury, or wound. Why does the sight of blood affect us so much? The reason is because it is the essence of life, the "lifeblood," and symbol of vitality.

Giver of Life

It is the woman who gives birth and passes on the gift of life. In former times women were seen as the only creators of life, dedicated to the creator goddess, and their monthly blood was sacred. During their period, they retreated into menstruation huts so that they could be with only women during this time. It was a kind of vacation because they were taken care of and didn't need to work. This would later be interpreted as though the women were excluded because they were "impure."

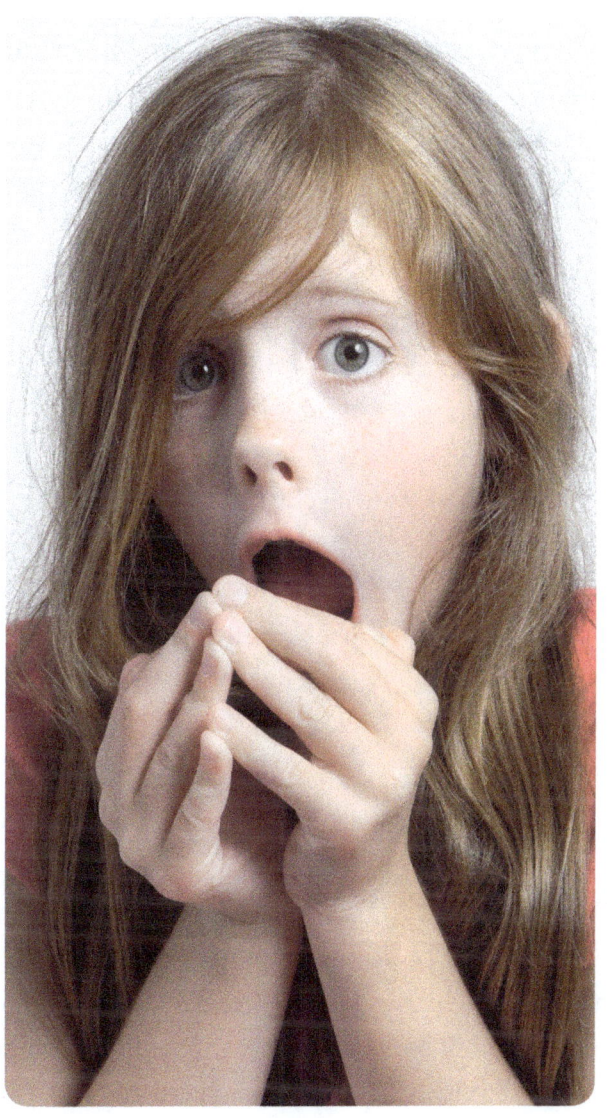

Most people are shocked when they see blood as it is often associated with injury and accident.

Blood signalizes something of the utmost importance, something mysterious, magical and unalterable. Important documents were written, and eternal friendships between two people were sealed with blood.

Causes of Bleeding Remained Unknown for a Long Time

This unique situation where blood flows without injury, without danger of bleeding too much and with no real wounds, is part of every woman's life; not just once, but again and again at regular intervals. If the body uses such a powerful signal then the message must be important; however, for a long time it couldn't be explained what this message was. Over the course of history different cultures tried to guess the reason for this mysterious occurrence.

Healing Nectar
In some cultures the menstrual blood was compared to the nectar of specific flowers. In India it was called "the nectar of the Kula flower." When young girls had their period it was said "the flower has come into blossom." Clothing materials were soaked in menstrual blood because they then possessed special healing power.

Blood is a Sign of Vitality and Power

Blood is a powerful symbol for strength which doesn't seem to match up with the assignment of women as the "weaker sex." If someone perceives a woman's vitality as a threat to his own power, he will try to weaken and devalue her in various different ways.

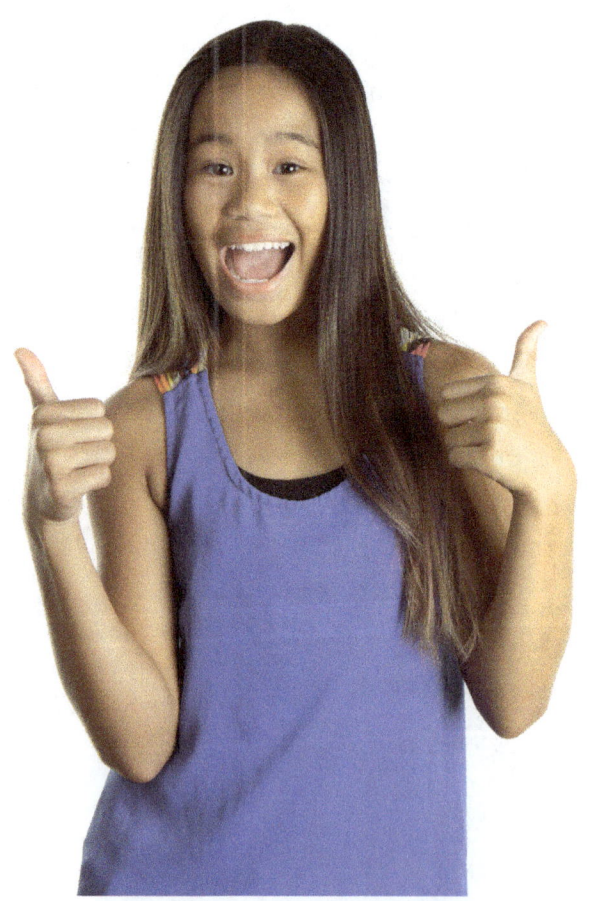

Things that frighten people are often made fun of in order to be able to deal with them. Unfortunately, these issues are still frequently found in our society today and have led to many prejudices that influence how menstruation is handled, and as a result, how much the woman herself is valued.

Is Nobody Allowed to Notice that you have your Period?

Menstrual bleeding is still hidden behind a wall of silence and considered one of the greatest taboos in our society. Women's self confidence still suffers from the fact that apparently something dirty and unclean is "down there." Showing a blood stain in public is associated with serious embarrassment. Pantyliners, sanitary pads, and tampons are freely advertised on prime-time television, but there is only one single aim with these ads, and that's to convey the message that no one should notice that you have your period! The sanitary products which are considered the best are those which achieve this perfectly. The red color of menstrual bleeding appears unacceptable according to advertisements, and blue blood apparently flows in women's veins. There isn't even any mention of the word "blood."

What's Really Happening in the Body

Dirty and Impure
In some cultures menstrual bleeding was previously considered to be impure and dirty. Women were excluded from "clean society" during their menstruation.

It is only in recent decades that people have been able to decipher what happens during the period. Guess work is a thing of the past, thankfully, as now everyone can and should know what is really going on in a woman's body.

Let's take a look at the Small Finale again. Since our body is wealthy and doesn't need to cut corners, it prepares the Luxury Suites anew every month. The top layer of the uterine lining has now become thick, soft, and very cozy. If the love letter to the corpus luteum fails to appear, consequently it becomes clear to the body that no guest has arrived. Then the nutrient packed uterine lining will not be saved and offered to the next guest. Everything is prepared again and again because the body can afford to do so.

Pure Luxury
The tiny blood vessels in the top layer of the uterine lining burst open and flush out the unused luxury. The gland cells, responsible for providing nutrients and immunity, and the walls and ceiling of the Luxury Suite are all washed away. The completely clean, nutrient rich blood flows out through the vagina, together with tissue fluid and small bits of mucus membrane. This process is a clear sign of how much power and energy is in your body.

Your period is also a great reminder for you to take care of yourself.

The Small Finale – Facts and Background

❀ *The period normally lasts between three to five days. The bleeding can be lighter or sometimes heavier.*

❀ *Roughly two thirds of the total amount of blood flows out in the first two days, the remaining third in the following days.*

❀ *Your period may sometimes seem heavy, but the total amount of blood is on average 2-3 fluid ounces. It's not normally difficult for the body to quickly regenerate this blood, but if a woman is experiencing very prolonged and heavy bleeding then in time anemia can occur.*

❀ *Menstrual blood doesn't clot like blood from a wound, it's not supposed to! Otherwise the lining of the womb couldn't be replaced, and the renovations couldn't take place. The Small Finale is an important part of the Cycle Show, and not a physical injury.*

❀ *The menstrual blood contains many nutrients: vitamins, proteins, sugar, iron, copper, magnesium, calcium, potassium, other mineral salts, and an abundance of antibodies.*

The Reason for this Abundance is Obvious:

The clearing out of the luxury hotel in your uterus is nothing more than the removal of the highly nutritious and unneeded cozy corners. It would have been possible for a new human being to grow there. The red blood cells would have supplied it with oxygen, the nutrients would have fed it, and the antibodies would have protected it from illnesses.

The menstrual blood is not dirty; it is completely clean and nourishing.

Different than Usual

The time before and during menstruation is not a particularly special time for many women; they continue life as usual.

For some, however, it is a phase in which they:

- Have a greater sense of smell
- Perceive colors more intensely
- Sense atmospheres better
- Feel affection more sensually
- See things more clearly
- Sense their female power and strength, but also their powerlessness
- Are much more in tune with the depths of their soul and the unconscious
- Develop more creativity and intuition
- Experience happiness and sadness more intensely

These are the days of "blood sisterhood" with your own body. They are your special days and your special time!

Like a Machine: Functioning the Same Every Day?

Your body is asking you to listen; with gentle pressure it is making its voice heard. The body's signs for this are tiredness, abdominal pain, headache, irritability, a feeling of tension, and mood swings. Instead of correctly interpreting this message, it is often completely misunderstood, and the menstrual bleeding looked upon as a "mishap of nature."

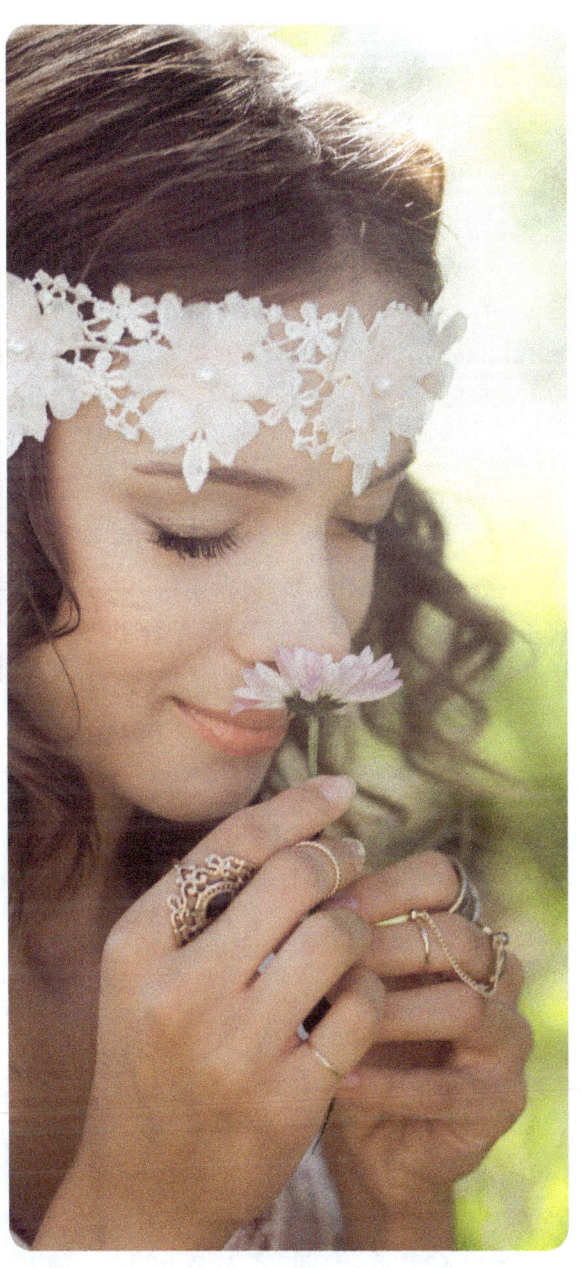

Some women have a more acute sense of smell during their period.

According to the expectations of society, during her period a woman is supposed to function just as smoothly as usual in school, training, and family life. Everyday life doesn't tolerate any drop in performance.

In this way, menstruation is made into a hygiene "problem." The focus is put on how each sanitary pad or tampon can be packaged and disposed of so that no one notices, and everything is managed cleanly and discretely. Tiredness, headaches, and abdominal pain are reduced to medical issues, which are to be cured by medication. Efficiency should not in any way be reduced.

Women's emotional outbursts before and during the period are seen as a case for the psychiatrist. When women recognize injustices and are no longer prepared to accept them, if they speak their minds openly, they are considered to be unstable, hysterical, and unpredictable.

Many women have already learned this false interpretation of our body language. During this time when they feel they are not meeting their own demands or those of others, they feel miserable, weak and restricted, and mourn their fate. The correct interpretation of this body code, however, is simply, "You are okay; please take care of yourself!"

The Thing about Period Pains

Naturally it's quite hard work for the body when the Luxury Suites in the uterine lining are removed and transported out. However, it doesn't necessarily have to be painful or cause discomfort. It's still not clear why some women have pain during their period while others don't. Or, why period pains end for many women after the birth of their first child and only begin then for others.

It is presumed that the different natural messenger substances (i.e the hormones: estrogen, progesterone, oxytocin, vasopressin, prostaglandins, and catecholamine) don't always interact harmoniously. This leads to the uterine muscle contracting painfully, similar to the contractions at birth, sometimes causing dizziness and nausea.

> *Many women were "pre-programmed" to equate the bleeding with burden, illness, and pain.*

But these hormonal factors are only one side of the coin, namely the physical one. There are other psychological and external reasons why some girls and women experience pain at varying levels and suffer so much with their period. This can lead to fears, tension, and spasms which only make the pain stronger.

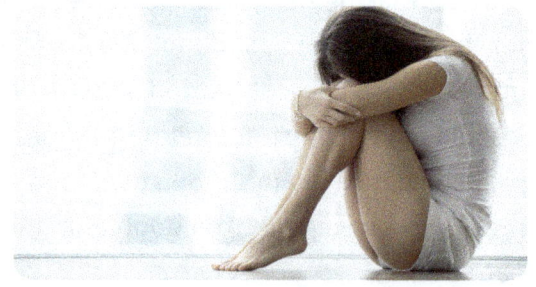

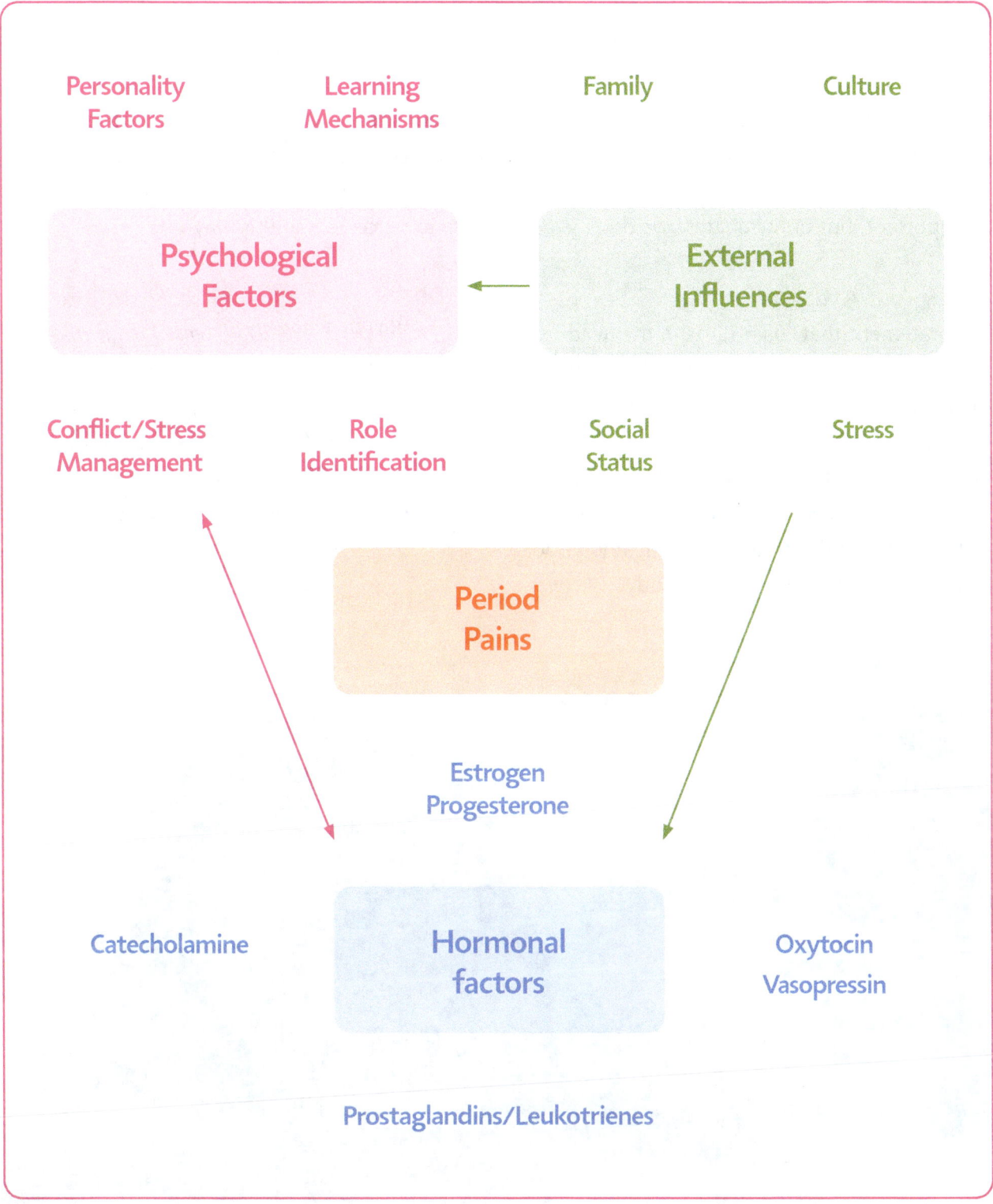

Menstrual problems can have many causes. In addition to physical reasons, psychological and external influences also play a role.

Make the Days of Your Period Special

Imagine that the period could be seen the same way in our society as a relaxing weekend following a strenuous school week, or as a day you come home with good grades for great achievement. Do you notice the positive feelings when you think about this? There is no doubt that the period is just as important, but unfortunately we don't yet seem able to perceive it in this way.

Check Your Attitude

The statement that "pain starts in the head" is admittedly not always true, but before you use medication, try a little self-love and care first.

Answer the question your body is asking you honestly. Do you like the way your body is and how it looks as a woman's body? To be loved is the basic foundation for wellbeing and good health; it's no different for your body.

Anyone who gets all tensed up at the beginning of the period is most likely to feel exactly the pain that was feared. This most commonly takes place unconsciously and is made worse by the seal of secrecy surrounding the event.

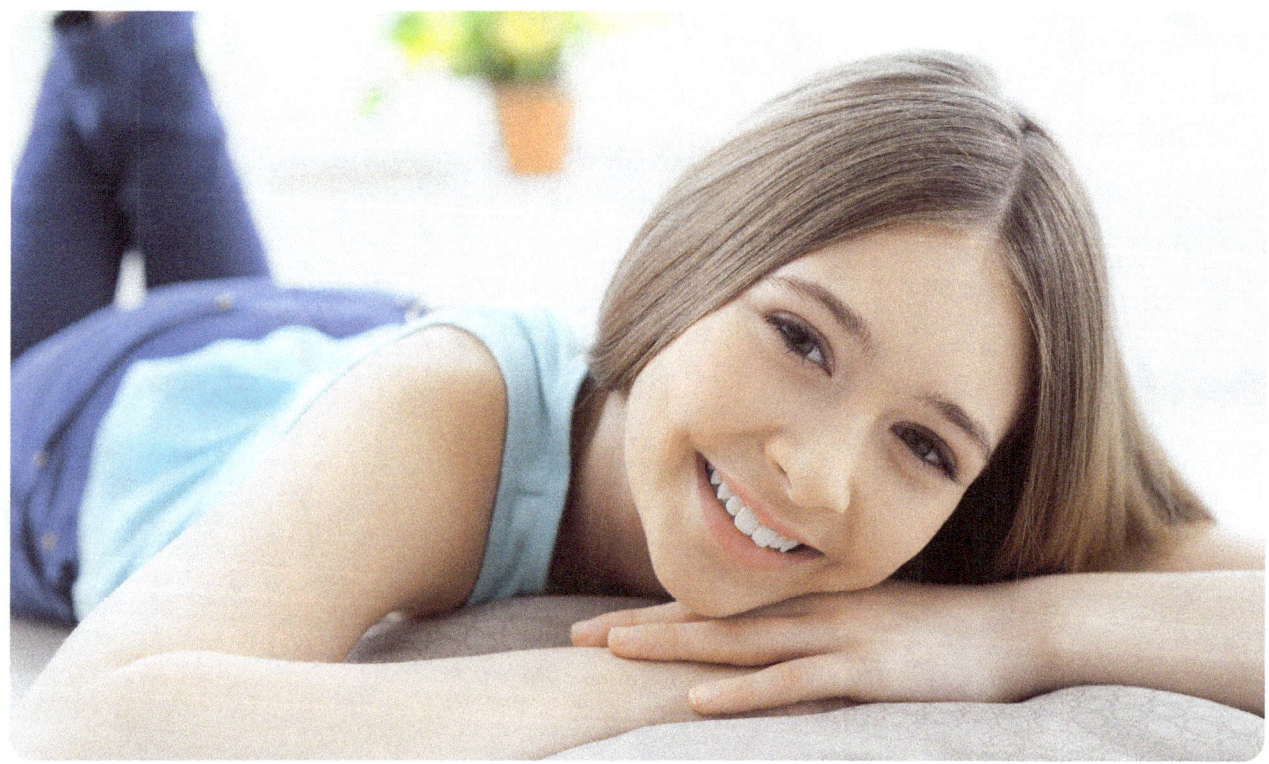

"Good days"

Begin to Reprogram!

Now that you know what's going on inside your body during the Cycle Show, the foundation to make these days special has been laid. Forget all the negative things you've ever heard about your period from now on. Positive thoughts are the next steps to feeling healthy.

A Few More Tips for Special Days:

- *Have a hot drink*

- *Do some exercise*

- *Take a nap*

- *Relax and make yourself comfortable with abdominal breathing, rocking with legs crossed and massaging the belly in a circular motion.*

- *Put a heat pack on your tummy.*

- *Read a captivating book or listen to nice music.*

- *It's perfectly okay if you require more peace and quiet, and you wish to be on your own.*

- *Take pain relief if needed. If your pain is severe, go and see your doctor.*

- *Be patient with yourself! In fact, be nicer to yourself than usual.*

Take care of yourself – these are your special days!

Sanitary Pads or Tampons – Whatever Suits You Best

Whether you wish to use sanitary pads or tampons during your period is entirely up to you. Most girls start with sanitary pads and don't try out tampons until later, when they are more familiar with their periods and know their bodies better. Many women manage well with sanitary pads all their life. They exist in all possible shapes and sizes: thick and thin, long and short, wide and narrow, with and without wings, in bulk packs or individually wrapped. Women who like pads appreciate the feeling that their blood can flow freely out of the vagina. All sanitary pads have an adhesive strip so they can be stuck securely to your underwear and a plastic film on the underside so the blood cannot soak through. Choose a product you feel happy with. You can share different products with your friend or your mother to try them out.

How often you change the pad depends on how heavy your bleeding is. The first few days you'll need to change it more often. After that, you may only need a new pad once or twice a day. You'll quickly find all this out for yourself.

The blood only begins to decompose when it comes into contact with the air. This can sometimes cause an unpleasant smell which can be avoided by changing the pads regularly. Always keep a small, well packaged pad in your school bag, even if you haven't started your period yet.

Greater Freedom with Tampons

Tampons are small rolls of very absorbent cotton wool, pressed tightly together with a small thread for removal. The tampon is inserted into the vagina with a finger or the help of an applicator if provided. Depending on the heaviness of the bleeding, it is pulled out after four to five hours during the day, and eight to nine hours at night. If the tampon is in the right position, you shouldn't feel it. It can be a slightly unpleasant feeling the very first time you try to use one. If you can still feel it inside, then you should push the tampon up a little further.

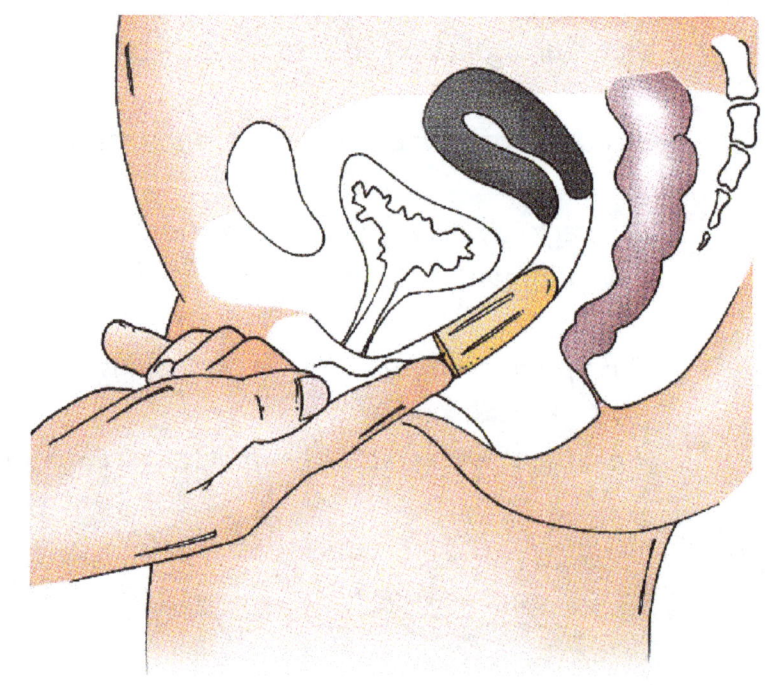

This is how to insert a tampon into the vagina.

> **By the way:**
> You don't need to remove the tampon when you go to the bathroom. The urine has its own outlet through the urethral opening, which lies in front of the entrance to the vagina.

Women and girls value tampons particularly because the blood is immediately caught in the vagina, and therefore they have more freedom to do what they want: swim, dance, ride, and cycle. (Caution: the tampon should be changed immediately after swimming).

The disadvantage of tampons is that they can dry out the vagina and possibly disturb the natural protective environment there. For this reason, they should only be used during the days when bleeding is at its heaviest. At night time, or if bleeding is heavy, you can use a pad in addition to the tampon so that the pad can absorb the blood if the tampon happens to overflow.

If your hymen is still intact, a small tampon should normally fit through the stretchy opening, and it shouldn't be a problem to remove it again. For some girls, for cultural reasons for example, it is very important that their hymen remains intact and therefore they should never be forced to use tampons.

> It's up to you to decide if and when you want to use a tampon. For example, no one should force you to take part in school swimming just because "everyone can use tampons nowadays."

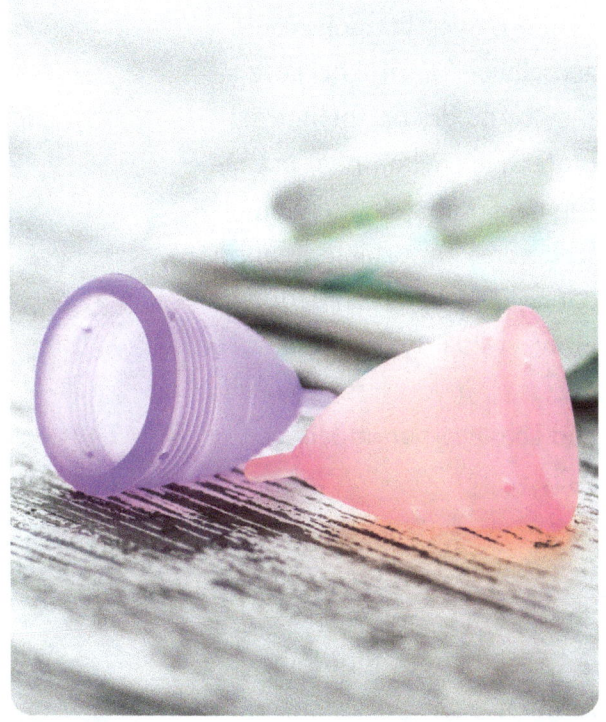

You can use sanitary pads, tampons, or menstrual cups, whatever you like.

An Alternative: Menstrual Cup or Washable Pads

Sanitary pads and tampons are disposable items which, over the years, create a huge amount of waste and cost a lot of money. Some women therefore wish to make use of reusable sanitary products for environmental protection and cost reasons.

Nowadays it is possible to buy different types of menstrual cups. This is a small silicon cup which is inserted into the vagina and put over the cervix to catch the blood. It is also possible to buy washable pads that can be reused.

Panty Liners – Not Really Necessary

You don't need sanitary pads or tampons when your period is over. Tampons could actually be harmful because they could dry up the normal protective environment in the vagina. Some girls and women feel more comfortable wearing panty liners between periods. However, panty liners are not necessary if you wash yourself and change your underwear daily.

Remember: The mucus which flows out of your vagina between periods is nothing less than a Magic Potion, completely hygienic and pure.

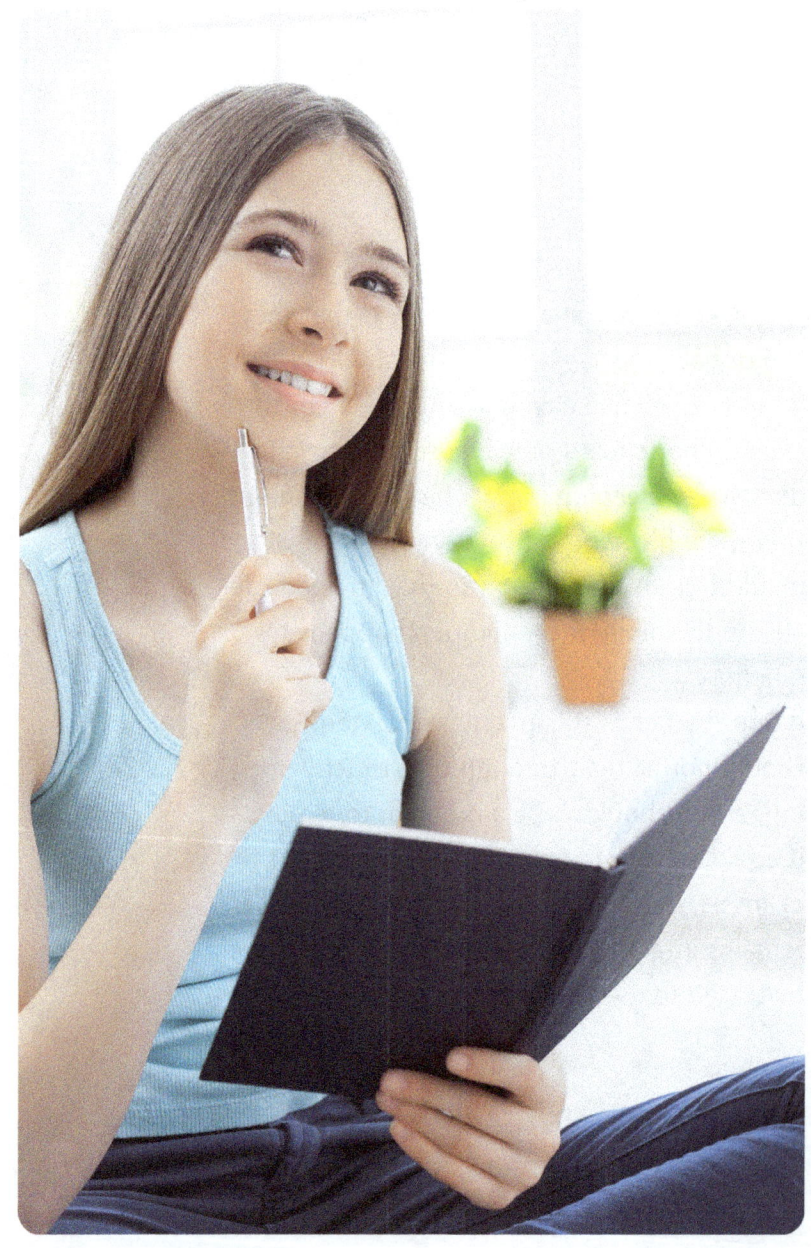

Anyone who regularly observes her body signals and enters them into a menstrual cycle diary will find out what is currently happening in the Cycle Show.

7 Looking for my Body's Secret Code

Observing the Physical Signs

Have you ever done a crossword puzzle? Completing the puzzle without the use of a pencil and paper and having to memorize the order of the words would be an impossible task. You answer the clues and then fill in the correct word, the more answers you get the more letters you have to help you complete the puzzle. In so doing, the whole thing gradually comes together. Our body language acts exactly the same way.

Only those who take note of its messages can crack the code and see the pattern emerging! By charting your observations, these patterns can quickly be seen. The red curtain is pushed aside, the spotlights switched on and you realize that this is the Cycle Show. The first act of the show is now playing live in your own body, which will be followed by the second act and finally the Small Finale. If you have the desire to discover your body and wish to see for yourself all that's taking place in it, then take the time to do so by listening to your body's messages. It's worth it!

The Cycle Show Chart Nowadays, instead of using pencil and paper, many girls and women record their cycle chart more easily on their mobile phone or computer. There are many apps available for download. These apps are useful to record and store your data, but do not rely on them to interpret your fertility. On the following pages you'll find extracts from Abigail's cycle chart. She is 15 years old and has been recording her daily body signals every evening for the last four cycles. The cycle days are already numbered consecutively and the respective date is underneath. On the top right you record the cycle number and that's it! Everything you noticed about your body and how you felt throughout the day can be entered into the chart every evening.

It Starts with the Small Finale Since the cycle events take place in a never ending circle, with no beginning and no end, the start was randomly selected. It was agreed that each cycle begins with the Small Finale. The first day of the period is also the first day of the cycle. A cycle lasts until the day before the next menstruation. Whenever a new period begins, a new page is started and a new cycle chart is begun.

MY CYCLE CHART

Thermometer: ☐ Oral ☐ Anal   Cycle No.: _____

Cycle day	1	2	3	4	5	6	7	8	9	10	11	12	13	14	15	16	17	18	19	20	21	22	23	24	25	26	27	28	29	30	31	32	33	34	35	36	37	38
Date																																						
How do I feel? 😊 😐 ☹ What's going on? Disturbances?																																						
My period																																						
Time of taking temp.																																						

BODY CODES — Looking for the progesterone temperature rise in my body

Temp																																						
37.2 °C																																						
37.1 °C																																						
37.0 °C																																						
36.9 °C																																						
36.8 °C																																						
36.7 °C																																						
36.6 °C																																						
36.5 °C																																						
36.4 °C																																						
36.3 °C																																						
36.2 °C																																						
36.1 °C																																						
36.0 °C																																						
Breast tenderness Ovulation pain																																						
Cervical mucus — M+																																						
M																																						
m																																						
d, Ø																																						
What's happening in my cycle?																																						

Looking for my Body's Secret Code

Abigail's Cycle Chart

In this cycle Abigail's period lasts for five days (see chart page 81). Bleeding was light on the first day, the second and third days were heaviest, and then it became lighter again. Abigail recorded the length and the heaviness of her period on her chart with small blood drops. She was also able to record how she felt during the cycle.

Body Code: Cervical Mucus – "Discharge" or a "Magic Potion"?

Unfortunately there are girls and women who have never heard anything about the most important secret code in their body. When they see or feel cervical mucus, they are afraid that they are ill because they have a discharge. Sometimes young girls are examined by a doctor before their first period because of this concern.

When girls and women discover mucus in their underwear or on the toilet paper, then their body is simply signaling that the first act of the Cycle Show is in progress! The eggs have been woken up and the estrogens are now on the move, having opened the season in the Leisure Center (in the cervical mucus glands). Girls who don't know this secret code are understandably often upset and possibly disgusted:

"Yuck, what's going on? Such strange stuff! What is happening to me? Am I ill? Is there something wrong? Where is this coming from?"

If you can decipher this body code correctly, you'll know that the cervical mucus is no strange discharge, it is the most important sign of female fertility.

> **FACT**
> *Discharge can actually arise if the lactic acid bacteria are unable to do their work properly in the vagina because they have been disrupted by incorrect hygiene practices (perfumed wipes, over washing or tampons used outside of the period), by medication (different antibiotics), or by hormonal contraceptive methods. The vaginal lining can become disturbed by bacteria or fungus. You will notice this by a feeling of itchiness, burning, and the presence of whitish, yellowish or greenish mucus, which may have an unpleasant smell. In this case you should see a doctor. The cervical mucus, however, has nothing to do with this discharge.*

Dry, Moist or Wet
Code I: Ever Noticed This Before?

You happen to be sitting on the commuter train or bus, doing homework or listening to music, when you suddenly have the sensation that something is trickling down the vagina. It feels like blood during your period and you are very conscious of it. On other occasions the vaginal area can feel moist, or even really wet.

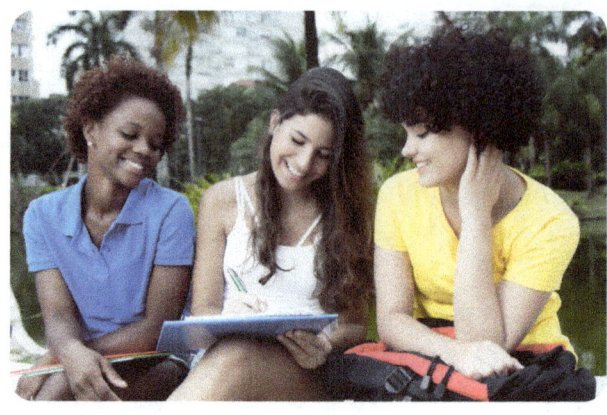

There are some days when there is no sensation at all, and yet on others the vagina can feel very dry and itchy, like when the skin on your hands is dry and in need of some moisturizing cream. In the same way that your rumbling tummy tells you

If you've learned to recognize the cervical mucus, then you become much more conscious of the sensations in the vaginal area throughout the day; such as: dry, nothing, moist, wet, etc.

that you are hungry and your dry mouth says you need something to drink, you will know exactly what's going on in your body if you recognize these body codes.

→ Dry or Felt Nothing

A dry feeling often occurs in the days directly following the period, and then again following ovulation in the second phase of the cycle. It tells us that no Estrogen Friends are busy at work; therefore the Magic Potion is either not yet or no longer available – which means bad times for the sperm!

→ Moist

This means pay attention, something is happening! The season is opening! The eggs are beginning to ripen in the ovaries, and the first Estrogen Friends have arrived at the cervical mucus glands and are starting to produce the Magic Potion. Should sperm appear on the scene, they already have a good chance of surviving in the Leisure Center at the cervix.

→ Wet

A wet sensation in the vaginal area means that your body is being pampered by a great number of Estrogen Friends. During this time an egg is getting ready in the ovaries to start its great adventure. There is plenty of cervical mucus, so the sperm would have a wonderful time!

TIP
Observe during the day and record it in your chart in the evening!

Dry or Slippery – Code II: Ever Tried to Feel It?

Everyone needs to go to the bathroom several times a day. And when you do, you wipe yourself with toilet paper. On some days the toilet paper slides over the vaginal opening like it was oiled, feeling much smoother and more slippery than usual. If you lightly brush your finger over it, the vaginal opening feels wet and slippery on those days.

→ Like It's Oiled

If on certain days you almost have the sensation of being "oiled" then you know exactly what's going on in your body at that moment. Lots of Estrogen Friends are busy, an egg is preparing for ovulation and the Magic Potion is in abundance. The sperm would find themselves in paradise!

Clumpy, Whitish or Clear – Code III: Ever Seen This?

You can really see the Magic Potion. It is present on certain days of the cycle and sticks to the toilet paper after wiping yourself. It changes in appearance depending on how many Estrogen Friends are currently at work. In this way, it is possible to keep track from the outside what is happening on the inside.

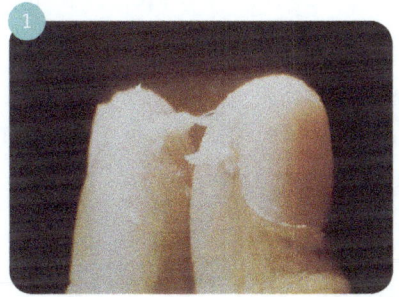
When you see the cervical mucus initially in the first phase of the cycle,

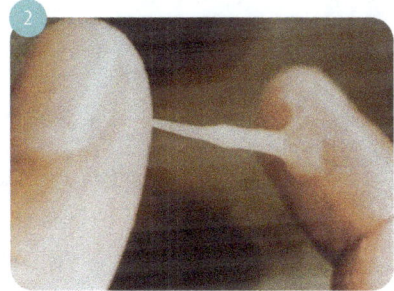
it is mostly whitish, thick and not very stretchy.

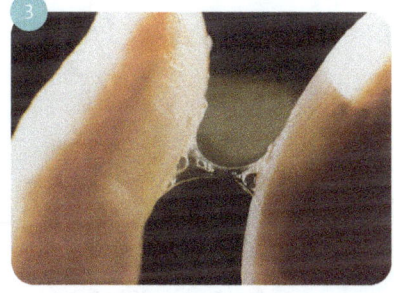
The more estrogens become active in the cervical mucus glands, the more transparent it becomes.

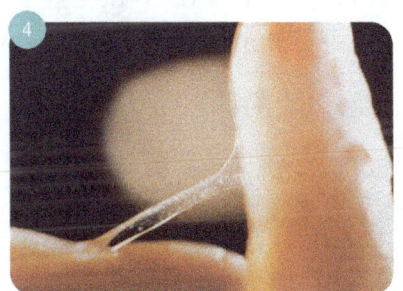
Around the time of ovulation it often looks like raw egg white.

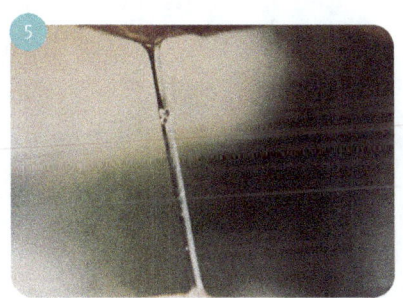
It can be stretched like a long thread.

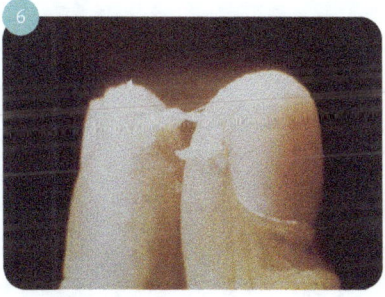
After ovulation, it quickly becomes thick once again and then disappears altogether.

→ Thick, Clumpy, Whitish

If you notice whitish, thick, sticky mucus for the first time in the course of the cycle, then the Estrogen Friends are at work. They've already produced so much Magic Potion that it spills out of the cervix, trickles down the vagina, and becomes clearly visible. In the ovary, an egg matures. The sperm could now spoil themselves for a few days in the Leisure Center at the cervix before being moved upwards in small groups to be in the right place when the time comes.

> **FACT**
> *Ovulation frequently takes place on the last day of stretchy, clear cervical mucus or the following day when little to no mucus can be seen or felt. It is not possible to pinpoint the exact moment of ovulation using your body's code. However, this is not necessary.*

→ Clear and Stretchy

Over the next days the cervical mucus increases, it becomes clear and looks like raw egg white. It gets stretchier and can hang out of the vagina in a long thread when you visit the toilet. It becomes even more liquid so that you have the sensation in the vaginal area of being really "wet". When all this happens, you know that a vast number of Estrogen Friends are very busy in your body, that ovulation could happen any minute, and the sperm could be having a wonderful time bathing in the Magic Potion.

> **FACT**
> *Don't worry if you have not seen any stretchy, clear cervical mucus yet. Every woman's mucus is different. Some women have never seen this stretchy, clear mucus and are still completely healthy. It is important however to notice the change in the quality of your mucus as it moves from fertility to infertility.*

→ All Gone

You suddenly notice the cervical mucus has disappeared, or has decreased, and is now only whitish and sticky. This tells you that the Ovulation Helpers have received their orders from the manager and the egg will now risk her adventurous jump. Any sperm present really must hurry if they are not to miss the next few crucial hours in which the egg is waiting for them. The fertile time is coming to an end.

Abigail's Cycle Chart

Following her period, Abigail couldn't feel anything at all in the vaginal area between the sixth and eighth days of the cycle. On the ninth day she had a "tingling" sensation in the vagina and it felt moist, so she recorded this in her cycle chart in the evening. The following day she noticed the Magic Potion on the toilet paper for the first time. It was thick, whitish and sticky and remained like this the following days. On day 16 the mucus looked clear for the first time and hung like a thread. The next day she noted that it was also stretchy and she felt very wet. It was suddenly different on day 18. In the evening she realized that she had seen a little whitish, thick cervical mucus only once during the day, and she didn't see or feel anything more after that.

♡ ✿ MY CYCLE CHART

Thermometer: ☐ Oral ☐ Anal   Cycle No.: _____

Cycle day / Date			1	2	3	4	5	6	7	8	9	10	11	12	13	14	15	16	17	18	19	20	21	22	23	24	25	26	27	28	29	30	31	32	33	34	35	36	37	38
BODY CODES	How do I feel? 😊😐☹ What's going on? Disturbances?																																								
	My period																																								
	Time of taking temp.																																								
	Looking for the progesterone temperature rise in my body	37.2 °C																																							
		37.1 °C																																							
		37.0 °C																																							
		36.9 °C																																							
		36.8 °C																																							
		36.7 °C																																							
		36.6 °C																																							
		36.5 °C																																							
		36.4 °C																																							
		36.3 °C																																							
		36.2 °C																																							
		36.1 °C																																							
		36.0 °C																																							
	Breast tenderness Ovulation pain																																								
	Cervical mucus	M+																				M+	M+																	
		M														M	M	M	M	M	M			M																
		m												m																										
		d, Ø									Ø	Ø	Ø											Ø	Ø															
	What's happening in my cycle?																																								

If you observe the cervical mucus you can use different abbreviations:

- **d** — dry sensation in the vaginal area
- **Ø** — felt nothing, saw nothing
- **m** — moist sensation in the vagina
- **M** — whitish, yellowish, thick, sticky, non-stretchy mucus
- **M+** — wet, slippery, clear, stretchy, like raw egg white

Body Code: Temperature Shift – The Progesterone Team Turn the Heat Up

We've already talked about the fact that following ovulation the central heating system in the brain is turned up by the Progesterone Team, which is produced by the corpus luteum. The temperature rises and we like to think this is because babies like to be warm. The woman's body temperature rises in the second phase of the cycle by about one degree fahrenheit. Obviously we don't feel this minimal heat rise,

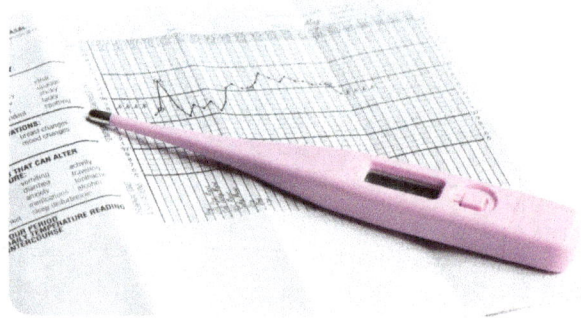

There are different thermometers available but not all are suitable for measuring the temperature rise caused by the progesterone.

you need a very precise measuring instrument and very exact measurement conditions to detect these gentle signals.

You should note the following:
- You can measure in different ways:
  - in the mouth (oral)
  - in the bottom (anal)
- You shouldn't change the method of measurement within one cycle.
- Important to know: measuring under the armpits or in the ear is much too inaccurate.
- If you are measuring orally make sure that the temperature probe is under the tongue, close to the small tongue band. The mouth must remain closed while measuring. Furthermore, you shouldn't talk or drink beforehand and needless to say, not smoke either.

Instructions for Successful Measurement
To determine the temperature rise caused by the progesterone, it is necessary to use a thermometer. You can use the ordinary, non-mercury, glass thermometers which are very accurate.

If you have a digital thermometer at home, be careful to keep measuring for three minutes after the beep so that this very slight difference in temperature can be accurately recorded. Most digital thermometers are only suitable for measuring fever and not really sensitive enough for the gentle progesterone heat. If possible, try and use a thermometer specifically designed for measuring this tiny rise in temperature (basal body temperature).

In the Mornings – Before the Day Begins

When you come in from playing a sport, you are naturally hot, your face is flushed and you have perspiration on your forehead. If you measured your temperature then it would certainly be higher than normal.

Exercise and physical activity increase the temperature considerably. If you wish to determine the gentle rise in temperature caused by progesterone, it would prove extremely difficult to do so following ten push-ups, a run or a shower. Therefore you should take your temperature under the same conditions every day, when your body is completely at rest. As this only occurs while sleeping, the rule is:

Take your temperature immediately upon waking up.

The Later It is, the Higher It is

Anyone who has ever had a fever knows that the temperature rises throughout the day. Human body temperature is at its lowest in the mornings, and increases during the day by less than 1/2 degree Fahrenheit. It's at its highest in the afternoon at about 3pm, after which it decreases.

If a woman measures her temperature at 6am on one day and at 10am the next day, then the temperature difference caused by this change in time could be exactly the same amount as the temperature shift caused by the progesterone. If this factor is not taken into account, it could be mistaken for the progesterone shift.

This is why women were advised in the past to set their alarm clock and measure their temperature at the same time, early every morning. Needless to say, that's quite an inconvenience and is not necessary. To determine the temperature rise caused by progesterone accurately, it is important that you **measure your temperature immediately upon waking up and recording the time.**

Laid-back, Lively or Both
Which Type are You?

It's also helpful to figure out what "temperature type" you are; there are lively and laid-back characters.

ARE YOU A LIVELY TYPE?

Lively characters also respond in other situations with temperature spikes, for example if they:

- Have gone to bed too late.
- Have slept badly or too little.
- Have eaten too much the evening before.
- Have danced and partied excessively.
- Have drunk more alcohol than usual.
- Are stressed.
- Are on vacation.
- Are unwell, have a cold or are taking medication.

Lively characters are always on the move and busy. If these girls or women sleep a bit longer, the temperature immediately takes a little leap and rises by half a degree Fahrenheit. This could be mistaken for a temperature shift caused by the progesterone, so it is necessary to figure out the cause of this unusual temperature spike.

> **ARE YOU A LAID BACK TYPE?**
>
> Of course the cool stay cool, disturbances leave them unaffected. They are sensitive to the progesterone heat and nothing else.

Such extremely distinctive characters very rarely exist. Some things make us react quicker, in other situations we remain cool. However, it is fascinating to work out which incidents "stir us up" and which ones "leave us cold."

It is therefore important to note all possible influences and peculiarities in the cycle chart!

These temperature variations are also called "disturbances" as they can either hide, or be mistaken for, the correct temperature rise. In the chart, they are put in brackets.

Cracking the Code: Looking for Ovulation

To crack the code in our body we need to:

❀ Successfully measure a distinct rise in temperature for three days above the previous six.

❀ Guarantee that no disturbances are involved.

❀ Make sure the cervical mucus can no longer be felt or seen.

Then we know that the second act of the Cycle Show has begun. The egg has dared to make the leap. The corpus luteum has developed out of the empty follicle, and created the Progesterone Team who are now on the move. They close the Gate of Life at the cervix and now set up the interior of the Luxury Suites. The Shutdown Agreement takes immediate effect as no further ovulation is allowed to take place until the end of the cycle.

Imagine a situation where sperm had been allowed to make an appearance in the Cycle Show. If one lucky sperm had successfully fertilized the egg, then an embryo could now be traveling to the uterus. If all goes well, the Grand Finale is in preparation.

However, if the sperm got the timing wrong, and appear on the Stage of Life now - in the second act of the Cycle Show - they have no chance of fulfilling their lifelong dream.

Abigail's Cycle Chart

Abigail bought herself a thermometer at the pharmacy. Now she can measure the effect of progesterone on her body's temperature. At the end of her period, from the sixth day of the cycle, she takes her temperature every morning immediately after waking up.

On day 7 of her cycle, Abigail overslept and didn't have time to take her temperature. Day 8 and 9 fall on a weekend, when she stays in bed longer. As a result she doesn't take her

FACT

Women who know their bodies and observe its signals can predict much more accurately when their period will start. When the cervical mucus disappears and the body temperature rises, they can expect their period about two weeks later.

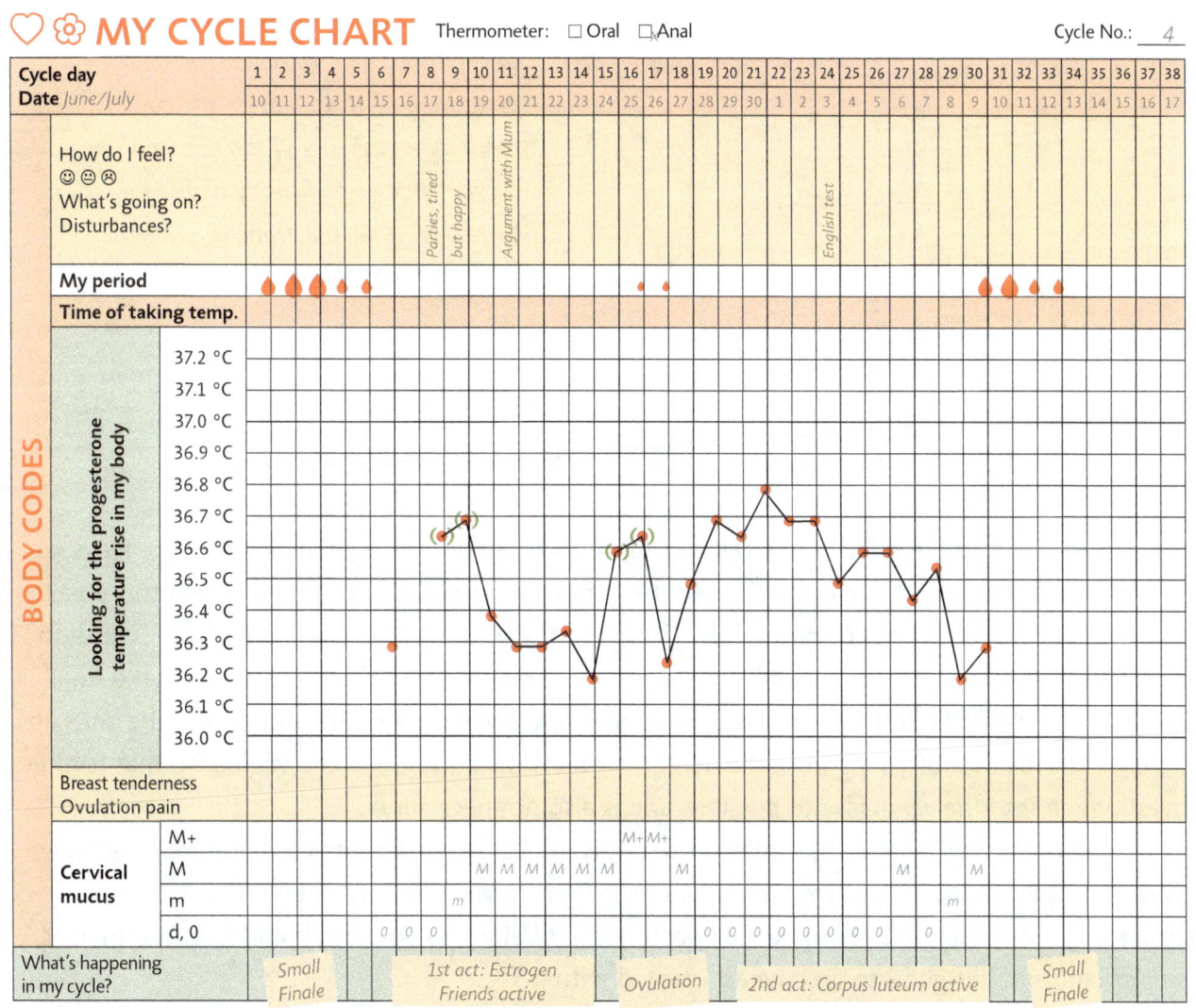

temperature until 10am and 11am, as she was at a party on Saturday evening. Her temperature takes a jump, but this doesn't bother Abigail because she knows it can't have anything to do with the progesterone rise.

The same thing occurs on day 15 and 16. Abigail just ignores the "disturbed values." The thermometer still doesn't indicate any progesterone rise. This is no wonder because Abigail observes a lot of cervical mucus in these days, a sign that the Estrogen Friends are still fully active and that ovulation has not yet happened.

On day 18 the temperature finally rises a little, less than half a degree Fahrenheit higher than on the past six days, apart from the disturbances. Abigail is curious about her next measurements. The temperature on days 19 and 20 is also higher than it was on the six previous days. Since the values were not disturbed and the Magic Potion has disappeared, she can assume on day 21 that the corpus luteum has now taken over. The second act of the Cycle Show has begun. Further measurements likewise reveal a higher temperature. After a total of twelve higher readings the Small Finale begins and with it a new Cycle Show.

> **FACT**
>
> *Unfortunately, it is not possible to see the exact day of ovulation from the temperature curve. Studies have shown that ovulation often takes place on one of the two days previous to the temperature shift, as well as on the day of the temperature rise. If the temperature curve remains significantly higher for three days, then one thing is for certain: ovulation is now over.*

Body Code: Cervix – The Gate of Life

This code is a little more difficult to crack and this may be an uninvestigated area for you. Have you ever looked at yourself "down below," seen the genital area with a mirror, and opened the labia? Have you ever touched your clitoris, which gives your body a very intensive, pleasurable sensation? Have you ever taken a look at the different entrances and exits belonging to your body: the small urethral opening at the front where the urine comes out, the vagina in the middle and the anus at the back? In the case of young girls, the hymen protects the entrance to the vagina, so that further investigation into the vagina is not possible, and is also not necessary.

Women who have already had intercourse or given birth to a child can continue to investigate inside their bodies and familiarize themselves with their cervix, the Gate of Life. This area, the entrance to your Stage of Life, is yours alone. It doesn't belong to your boyfriend, your partner, or your doctor, and it is good to become acquainted with it.

The Vagina – the Entrance Hall to the Stage of Life

Many different scenarios take place in the vagina. During menstruation, the pure luxury from the renovation of the Luxury Suites passes through on its way out of the body.

During the most intimate and beautiful drama between a woman and a man, full of love, desire and affection, the man's penis can slide into the vagina and the man has an ejaculation. If the timing is right, the sperm will meet the Magic Potion here and be admitted through the Gate of Life.

Ultimately, in the Grand Finale, the vagina again becomes the scene for a deeply moving event: a child will make its way into the world through the widened opening of both the cervix and the vagina.

Investigating the Cervix

If a women wishes to investigate the cervix, she inserts one or two clean fingers into the vagina. By sliding them diagonally towards the back and then upwards she initially feels the small "rippled" folds of the vaginal walls. If her fingers encounter a smooth, rounded surface, they have discovered the cervix. If she is not sure whether she has found it or not, then she hasn't felt it yet. Smooth and soft like the surface of a plump black cherry, it stands out against the folds of the vaginal wall. This sense of touch is totally unique. The opening to the cervix, which feels like a dimple, can also be discovered at the end.

Women who wish to observe the changes at the cervix should check it regularly, for example, every evening before going to bed. This is the best way to detect the minor changes in the first phase of the cycle. By contrast, the more dramatic changes of the cervix at the start of the second phase of the cycle are easier to observe.

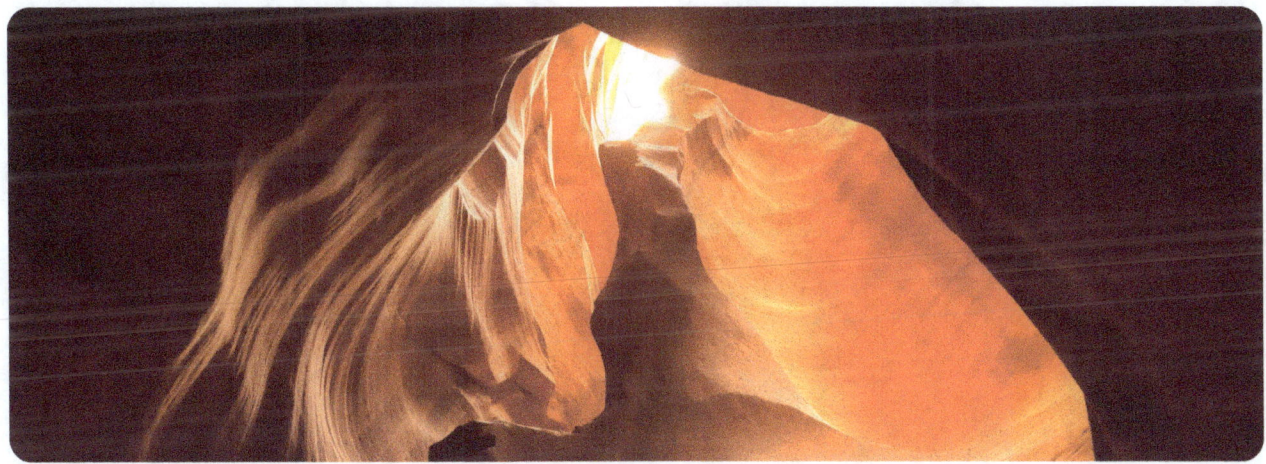

Investigating your own body can be as exciting as a magnificent natural spectacle.

→ Quite Firm

The Gate of Life changes depending on which act of the Cycle Show is currently playing. The cervix is slightly open during menstruation. Until the first Estrogen Friends arrive, the cervix feels firm, like the tip of the nose. The opening is quite small, as the Gate of Life is still closed.

→ Getting Softer

As soon as the Estrogen Friends start their preparations on the Stage of Life, they come to the cervix. Little by little, day after day, it opens its gates a little further. It becomes softer due to an increased blood supply, and feels similar to lips.

→ High Up and Open

In some women, the whole uterus stretches upwards, in joyful anticipation, so that it is scarcely possible at this time to feel the cervix with your fingers, and sometimes it's not possible to reach it at all. The cervix is very soft and opens to its widest (roughly .2 to .3 inches) at the time of ovulation, and cervical mucus flows out.

→ Closed Again

After a while, the corpus luteum resumes work with the Progesterone Team in the second act of the Cycle Show, and everything quickly reverts back. There is no point in keeping the gate open for new sperm; after all, the egg is either already fertilized or no longer alive. The cervix becomes firmer, closes up, and is now easier to reach again with the finger.

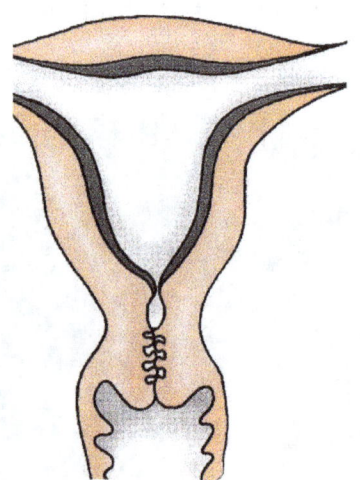

Following menstruation the cervix is closed, feels firmer, and can be reached quite easily.

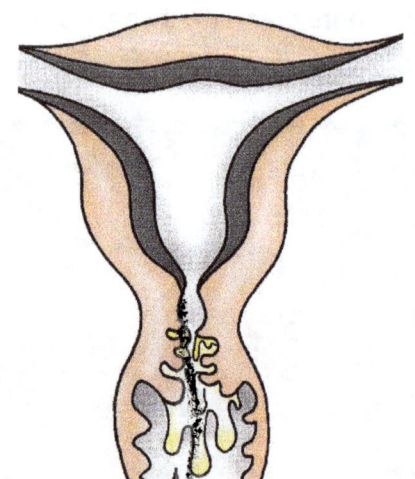

When ovulation is approaching it is soft, open, and more difficult to reach.

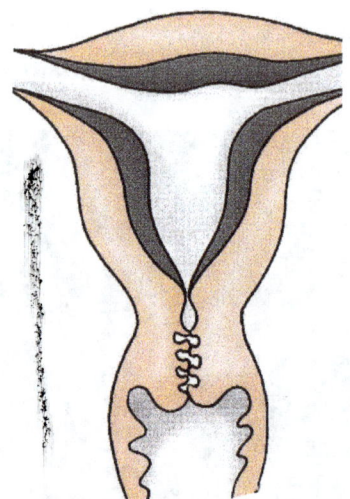

In the second phase of the cycle it is closed again and easier to reach once more.

Body Code: Ovulation Pain – Happiness can Sometimes Hurt

Perhaps you know that the feelings of happiness and pain are often quite closely related. Labor pains lead to the joyful occasion of birth. When someone is really looking forward to something, often just thinking about it hurts. It's the same with our body. The growth of a new egg and the prospect of "its birth" is an exciting event. The Estrogen Friends rush around the body announcing this great news.

> **FACT**
>
> *If a woman wishes to have a child and she has ovulation pain, then she should know that this is the best time to become pregnant. However, one shouldn't depend on ovulation pain as a form of preventing pregnancy.*

Strong Movement of the Fallopian Tube
The fallopian tube can scarcely wait to receive the egg when it takes the leap; it moves about as it tries to place itself over the growing follicle in order to catch the egg. These movements are caused by contractions of fine muscles due to a high level of estrogen at this time. These contractions could be one reason why some women feel abdominal cramps. New research suggests that another reason women notice pain on one side could be because of muscle contractions of the fallopian tube on the side where the ovulation will take place, sucking sperm into the tube.

"Totally Excited"
The follicle itself is also "excited." As it gets bigger and bigger and the tension starts to grow inside the increasingly thin bubble, it can sometimes feel almost unbearable and can cause the woman quite unpleasant pain.

Liquid on the Peritoneum
Occasionally it also hurts when the egg has taken its adventurous leap and a little liquid from the follicle runs down into the abdominal cavity. The very sensitive peritoneum reacts in its own way to the joyful message from above.

Not to Be Confused with an Appendix!
Only three in ten women experience ovulation pain (Mittelschmerz). When women notice this symptom for the first time, and suddenly feel strong twinges or cramp-like pains, they often don't know what it means. The problem is that these boisterous body signals could be misinterpreted as a

medical condition. It is therefore not uncommon that young women are concerned about this and go to the doctor. Sometimes it's not easy to decipher whether an acute abdominal pain stems from appendicitis or from harmless ovulation pain. Occasionally another misdiagnosis of "acute ovarian inflammation" is made and a completely unnecessary treatment carried out. The correct interpretation of the code is:

If you feel
- cramping, sharp or burning pain
- in the lower abdomen or on your left or right side
- either briefly or for up to a couple of days

there is no need to worry as long as cervical mucus is present at this time.

It will be clear to you that we're just dealing with ovulation pain; your body's feeling of happiness which sometimes hurts. Countless Estrogen Friends are now active and an egg is ready to take the leap from the ovary.

Abigail's Cycle Chart
On day 16 of this cycle, Abigail felt a couple of acute twinges in her right lower abdomen. Was that ovulation pain? She records the happening right away on her chart, just in case.

Body Code: Ovulation Bleeding – A Little Blood around the Time of Ovulation

Ovulation bleeding is also called intermenstrual bleeding; it happens around the time of ovulation and has nothing to do with the period. It is a rare occurrence, just like the ovulation pain, and unfortunately little is known about what causes it. We already mentioned that having triggered the brain to put the "Ovulation Helpers" (LH) into action, the Estrogen Friends withdraw for the time being and as a result the estrogen level drops. It is assumed that not enough estrogens are then active to adequately care for the top "floors" of the uterine lining, causing the top layer of the uterine lining to bleed slightly. But you have no need to worry, as you are able to decipher this code.

Abigail's Cycle Chart
Abigail is one of the young women who discovers a small amount of blood in her underwear at the same time the cervical mucus is present. Sometimes the mucus is a bit bloody and looks reddish. Only very occasionally is the bleeding heavier, so normally it cannot be confused with the Small

Finale. In this cycle, Abigail's cervical mucus has a brownish, or rather reddish color on day 16 and 17. That doesn't worry her, so she just notes it in her cycle chart.

Body Code: Breast Symptom – The Overeager Progesterone Team

Do you remember the overeager Progesterone Team that prepares the mammary glands in advance for breastfeeding a baby? They increase the blood supply to the breasts, causing the lobes of the mammary glands to develop. The best baby food in the world is to be produced here. As a result, in the second phase of the cycle, the breasts are often heavier and larger, they feel tighter, they are more sensitive to touch, and sometimes they're even quite painful.

FACT

Any other bleeding that occurs between periods and not around the time of ovulation should be discussed with a doctor. This rarely happens in young girls.

Under the light microscope, the progesterone from the corpus luteum appears to be like a luminous crystal.

Some women only feel this tenderness a few days before their period. Others notice it as soon as the Progesterone Team reach the mammary glands from the corpus luteum.

Every woman that has cracked this code understands that when her breasts tighten and become more sensitive to the touch, it has nothing to do with illness, let alone cancer, but merely with the overeagerness of the Progesterone Team. The second act of the Cycle Show is well underway and the Small Finale will begin within a matter of days.

However, if the sperm were in the right place at the right time a few days earlier in order to meet the egg, then the Grand Finale could lie ahead. Many women know this sign and say "Suddenly my breasts increased in size and got heavier. I knew I was pregnant!"

Abigail's Cycle Chart
Abigail's breasts become very tender to touch the final week before her next period. She almost has the feeling that her bra doesn't fit any more. She records this observation every day in her chart with a "B."

> **FACT**
>
> *There are still a lot of uncertainties concerning the true cause of the breast symptom. There is a strong case to be made for hormonal imbalance. There are currently even possible indications that suggest it could have something to do with a lack of progesterone.*

More Body Codes – Entirely Individual

There are a number of other less noticeable body codes. These are individual symptoms which can be connected to the Cycle Show, but don't have to be! While some women feel consistently well throughout the whole cycle, others are more sensitive and experience the change of the inner seasons very intensively, often experiencing various physical and emotional changes.

The Mood is Mostly Bright
Particularly in the first phase of the cycle, women tend to be in a good mood; they feel well, are full of energy, and are able to tackle a huge amount of work. They feel as if they could move mountains. Obviously, it's their abundance of Estrogen Friends that support them so well. Their skin is velvety and clear; their hair shiny; they feel good about themselves and enjoy life.

ALEX (13)
My mom often suffers from headaches, which make her unbearable. Leaving her in peace, as much as possible, is the best way for us to deal with it. She says she always gets them before her period. I hope that won't happen to me. Not everyone gets them. My friend's mom for example has no problems with that at all. No one even notices when she has her period.

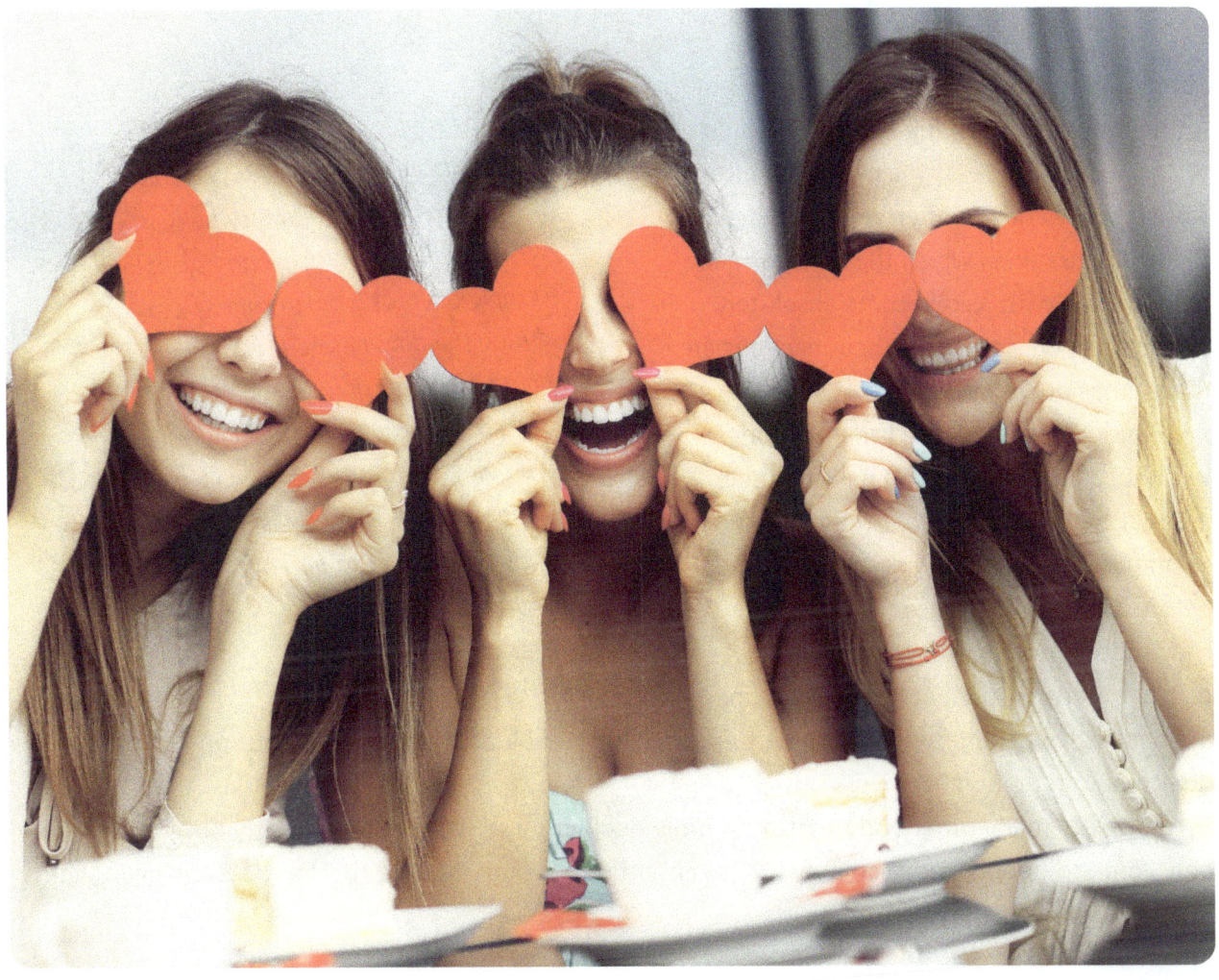

The Estrogen Friends ensure that you have a sense of wellbeing and that you're in good shape.

Some women notice that at certain times they desire more tenderness, and they also wish to allow the sperm to play their role in the Cycle Show. This feeling can occur during the time of menstruation, or in the first phase of the cycle when lots of Estrogen Friends are underway. Sometimes girls and women simply feel "in love" without knowing with whom or why, and long for love and tenderness.

The women who experience spring and summer very intensively in their cycle are naturally also the ones who feel the accompanying symptoms of autumn and winter more than others.

Feeling Down on Certain Days

Some women feel tired, worn out, and not in the mood for anything towards the end of the second phase of the cycle. Some can feel very low and are often close to tears. Difficult situations, which they are normally able to cope with, can become absolutely unbearable. Consequently their reactions are more emotional than usual.

Physically, some feel a little off-color, with outbreaks of acne and hair that gets greasier more quickly and is more difficult to manage than usual. Particularly just before the next period, some women get headaches or migraines, while others get diarrhea, constipation, or have the feeling of constantly needing to go to the bathroom. Some feel bloated and actually put on a few pounds due to fluid retention.

There are many other body signs that individual girls and women consistently observe, but they only come to understand them when they enter them into their cycle chart and recognize in which phase of the cycle they occur.

Something to Remember:
Many things that are blamed on a woman, often in a negative way, have nothing to do with the different emotional changes during the Cycle Show. For example, you may hear comments such as "don't mind her it's that time of the month." On the contrary, it is the normal daily situations that can give a girl or a woman a boost, or can drag them down. Women don't simply react like robots to both the sunny and dark sides of life, but with normal human feelings.

The easiest way to determine if and how the cycle affects a woman's life is to keep a cycle chart.

> **FACT**
> *Perhaps you've already heard about premenstrual syndrome (PMS). This medical term is like a "messy box" in which we store all the physical and psychological complaints that women suffer from during the days before their periods. There are so many possible reasons for PMS and nobody knows the real causes of the many disruptions to a women's well being. Medical science has not taken the trouble yet to try to find out.*

8 Cycle Length and Cycle Variation – When Am I Fertile?

What Exactly Do We Mean by Regular?

How long should a cycle be? We've been taught that a healthy cycle is 28 days long, so great care was taken when "the pill" was developed in order for it to replicate this four-week rhythm. It was intended to make women feel as though their bodies and cycles were, regular, healthy, and functioning normally. Many girls and women do have regular 28 day cycles; however, very few of them know that this supposed regularity has nothing to do with the events in their body.

Practice Required: Cycle Regulation during the First Years after the Menarche

Although it is well known that the cycle takes some time to regulate in the first few years following the first period, many girls become impatient and upset if their period is not yet regular. An analogy to this would be a mother going to a counseling center because her baby can only take one step and then falls down; occasionally he manages to take two but then falls again. The mother feels frustrated as he has been practicing for two days but is not able to walk yet! The reaction to this mother's impatience is easy to imagine.

When it comes to the rehearsals for the Cycle Show many react just as impatiently and illogically, expecting everything to run perfectly and regularly from the first period onwards. This doesn't happen, and it doesn't have to happen. Similar to real life, the first few years following the premiere require a

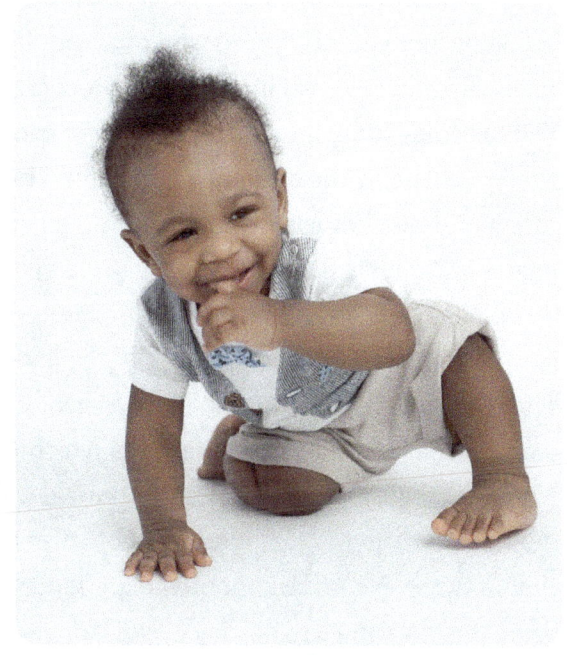

No expert has been trained in a day. The cycle also starts with "baby steps."

lot of practice and rehearsal.

There are many different variations in the practice phase of the Cycle Show. The phase up to ovulation is often extended, or the phase afterwards shortened, or both. It's quite common for ovulation to be left out altogether. This is all part of the official training program. All your body is asking for is for you to give it time and have a little patience with it.

> **FACT**
> *Some girls go to the doctor because of their "irregular cycle" and are given the COC pill (combined oral contraceptive pill), also known as the birth control pill, in order to "regulate the cycle." In doing so, their cycle is not regulated as a result, but in fact the whole program is completely cancelled and replaced by the artificial 28 day rhythm of the pill. If girls realized exactly what this entailed, would they really want to do it?*

Nothing Surprises Me Anymore!

It's understandable why women find it unpleasant to not be able to count on when their next period will arrive; they don't want it to come as a surprise or inconvenient time because that would prevent them from being able to plan or calculate anything. Women who are comfortable with their cycle and are familiar with their body codes don't experience this feeling of helplessness, as, despite possible irregularities, they know where they stand and when their next period is due.

Whether you're a young girl or an adult woman the same applies to everyone: the Cycle Show takes place live, in real life! It's not a recording. Good show hosts and actors don't stick stubbornly to their lines; they are flexible and react spontaneously to current events, taking their cue from their guests and the audience's reaction. This is what makes a show exciting and unique! The thrill of a live show, however doesn't fit into a predetermined broadcasting time, only pre-recordings last exactly 28 days.

Who Still Believes in the 28 Day Fairy Tale?

The reality is that no woman has cycles of exactly the same length for a whole year. Very few women (i.e. 3%) have cycle lengths which only vary by three days and always have cycles of just 27, 28, and 29 days. In most cases there is variety and diversity; sometimes a cycle lasts 27 days, the next 29 and the next 33. Out of 100 women, 60 have cycle lengths that vary in one year by more than a week. Nearly 1:2 women experience cycle irregularities of more than two weeks within one year; this means 26 to 40 day cycles, for example. Now that's what we call a live show!

So the "normal" 28 day cycle is not so normal at all. When the cycles of 10,000 healthy women were counted there was a surprising discovery; only 13% lasted 28 days. The frontrunner was the 27 day cycle, with no more than 14% of women. Longer cycles are much more common than shorter ones, almost half of the cycles (i.e. 45%) are longer than 28 days.

> **FACT**
> The normal life of a cycle takes place within a time frame of 23 to 35 days. Every now and again, there are shorter or longer "outliers" in between.

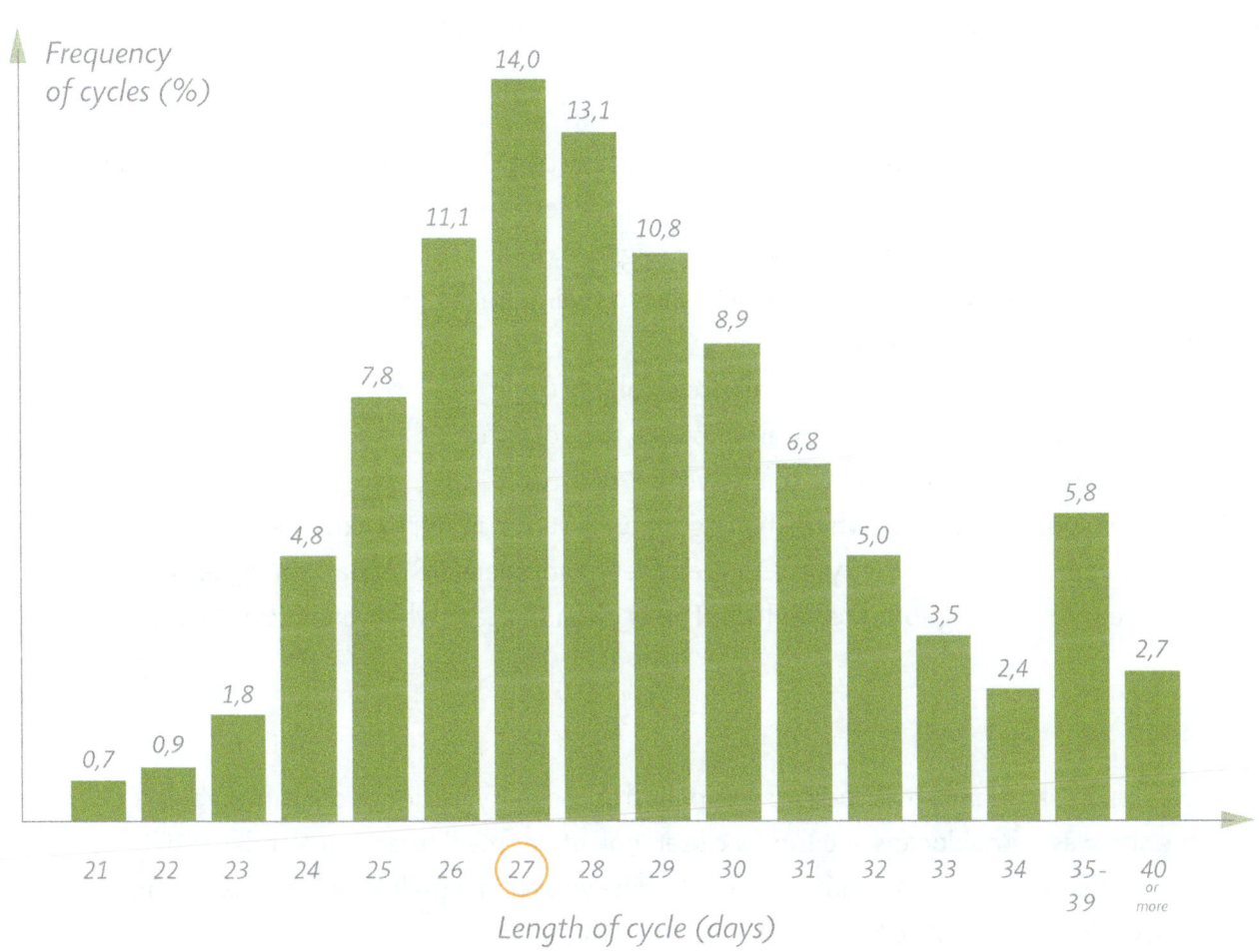

This analysis of 10,000 cycles shows the different cycle lengths of healthy women and how often they occur.

The First Act Varies, the Second is Constant

Sometimes the Cycle Show is mistaken for a football game, as it has two halves and a break in the middle. In many textbooks, and even in specialized medical literature, we often read that the classical 28 day cycle has two "halves" and that ovulation normally takes place on the 14th day. The reality is rather different, as this classic cycle rarely exists; therefore, it shouldn't be regarded as the standard.

> **FACT**
> *The first phase of the cycle varies in length. It can last for several days, but also for several weeks.*

It is correct that the cycle has two phases and that ovulation occurs at the transition from one phase to the other; however, both phases are rarely the same length.

Follicular Phase – First Phase of the Cycle: Sometimes Longer, Sometimes Shorter

It is in the first phase of the cycle where the variability occurs. The duration of time required for the different activities varies. It depends on how long is needed:
- For the Messengers of Spring to wake the eggs.
- For the estrogens to form on the follicle and to swarm out to prepare the Stage of Life
    - To build up the uterine lining.
    - To open the cervix and produce the cervical mucus.
- For an egg to be chosen and prepared to take the adventurous leap.

This can take from several days to many weeks.

There are "sprinter" cycles in which the egg matures very quickly; in extreme cases, ovulation can occur as early as day 7 of the cycle. On the other hand, there are "marathon" cycles where it can take weeks for the egg to make the leap. This is often the case when the Cycle Show is still in

> **CORINNA (15)**
> "My older sister claims that she gets her period as regularly as clockwork, however last time she was at the doctors she took a closer look at her menstruation calendar and it showed that her cycles were not very regular. She even had a cycle of 42 days last summer but she didn't even notice because she was on vacation."

the practice phase at puberty or if a woman is under a lot of stress, has just stopped taking hormonal contraceptives or is going through menopause. Women who are familiar with their body language will still know which act is currently playing, as this can be detected by the body codes. When the cervical mucus suddenly disappears and the body temperature rises at the same time, she knows ovulation has taken place.

> **FACT**
> When the cervical mucus has either decreased or disappeared and the temperature has risen, the woman can expect her next period in 10 to 16 days. Women who don't observe their cycle only know when their ovulation took place once their period has started, i.e. 10 to 16 days before.

The Second Act: the Calming Influence

In comparison to the first act, the second act of the Cycle Show following ovulation is a quiet time. The corpus luteum is formed and the Progesterone Team go about setting up the luxurious uterine lining, closing the cervix, ending the production of cervical mucus and raising the body temperature. The preparation of the mammary glands begins and the Shut down Agreement is activated, just in case a fertilized egg is on its way to the uterus. After about one week, if the corpus luteum hasn't received any news, it will withdraw the Progesterone Team from the uterine lining. The next period will begin around two weeks after ovulation, or more precisely 10 to 16 days after.

When Am I Fertile?

The question of cycle length is not just about anticipating when the next period comes; it also changes the time in which a woman may become pregnant, her so called "fertile days." If people are asked when they think a woman is fertile, they commonly answer "mid-cycle" or "around day 14." If someone has a little more knowledge of the survival time of the sperm, they may say "between day 10 and 16." That is roughly what we learned at school; sometimes it is correct, but often it is not, so that knowledge turns into a problematic half truth.

Those who speak of the "mid-cycle" assume a woman has a 28 day cycle and that ovulation would occur around day 14. As this only happens in 13% of cycles, it can have serious consequences:

- Some couples will fail to get pregnant because they only try around day 14.
- Others will get pregnant when they don't want to, because they think that there are only a few unsafe days in the middle of the cycle.

The Fertile Phase

A woman can become pregnant five days before ovulation and on the actual day of ovulation. The fertile days include the three-to five-day lifespan of the sperm and the maximum one-day lifespan of the egg, meaning six days in all. This is called the "fertile window."

> **JASMIN (12)**
> "Recently I heard my mother telling a friend that she became pregnant with my brother on the seventh day of her cycle, at a time when her period was coming to an end. She thought that nothing could happen yet!"

Early Ovulation – Earlier Fertile Days

Many people think they are safe during the menstrual period and for a couple of days after (day 6 to day 9 of the cycle), but that's not always true. There are cycles in which the egg matures very rapidly. In 5% of cycles, ovulation takes place before day 12 of the cycle, and in 20% before day 14; in such cases the Messengers of Spring have already woken the eggs during menstruation and the estrogens rush to their places of work. It can happen that the first cervical mucus has already appeared during the last days of menstrual bleeding. We know that the sperm can survive in the mucus for up to five days, so it is possible that a woman may already be fertile during the last days of her period.

Correction:

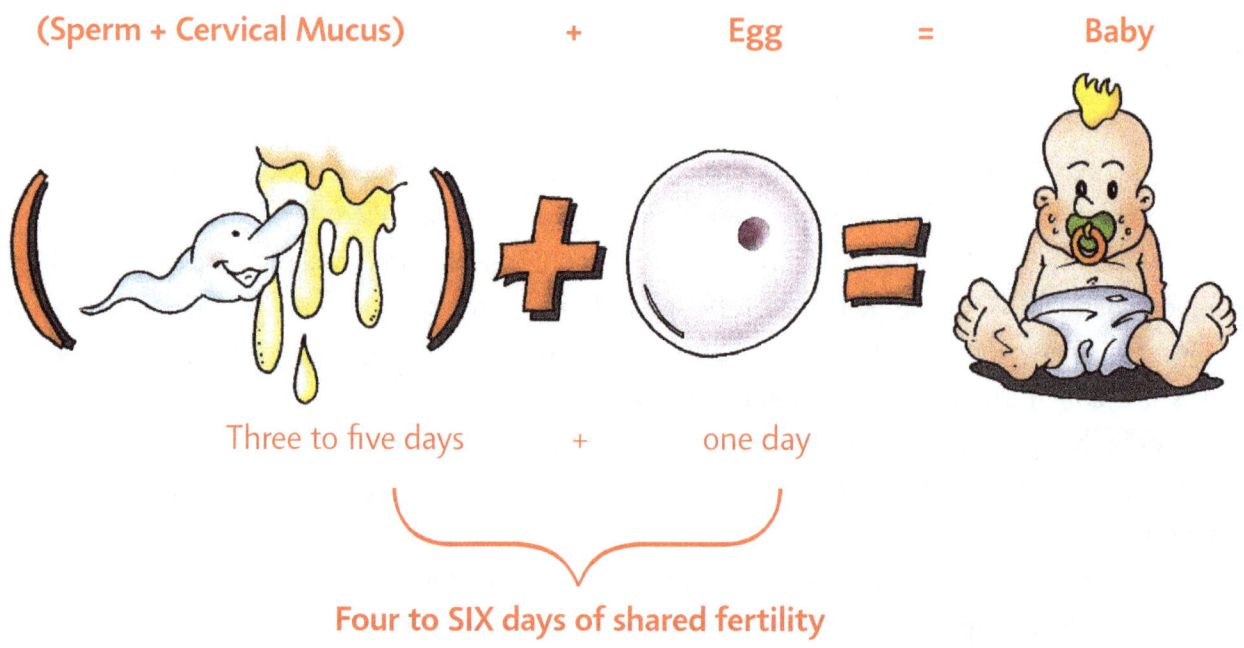

(Sperm + Cervical Mucus)   +   Egg   =   Baby

Three to five days   +   one day

Four to SIX days of shared fertility between a man and a woman in one cycle.

FACT

Be careful with using "fertility apps". Many are like a diary or calendar; they just record the dates of the menstrual cycle and do not try to predict the fertile and infertile phases of the menstrual cycle. They can be really helpful. Others attempt to predict the fertile phase only through calculation; nevertheless, you should not rely on this as pregnancy can result from an incorrect estimate of the onset of fertility.

FACT

- In over half of all cycles ovulation takes place after day 14.
- In 20% of all cycles ovulation takes place on day 20 or later.
- Among young girls and women ovulation often takes place even later than this.

(From a statistic of 10,000 cycles of healthy women.)

FACT

For women who don't know their cycle, every day of the cycle must be considered possibly fertile.

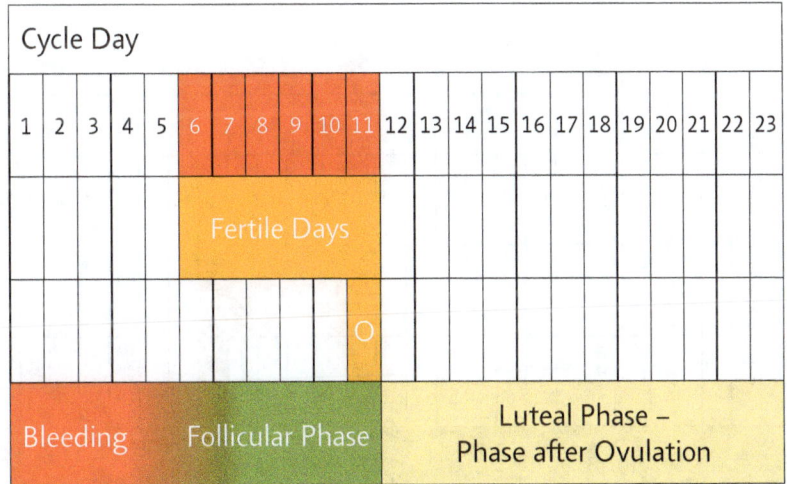

23 Day Cycle with Early Ovulation on Day 11

O = Ovulation

Late Ovulation – Later Fertile Days

The length of time it takes for an egg to mature until ovulation can be delayed; this in turn delays the fertile days. For instance, there can be "marathon" cycles where ovulation occurs ten weeks after the cycle began. Many women take a pregnancy test if their period doesn't come at the expected time. If the test is negative, they assume not only that they are not pregnant but also that they are no longer fertile because the cycle has gone on so long. This mistake can lead to unplanned pregnancies.

Women who observe their bodies will know what's going on in such cases. They will see that the follicular phase has simply been extended. So if planning a child, they will still be able to recognize their fertile phase, even if delayed by weeks.

35 Day Cycle with Late Ovulation on Day 23

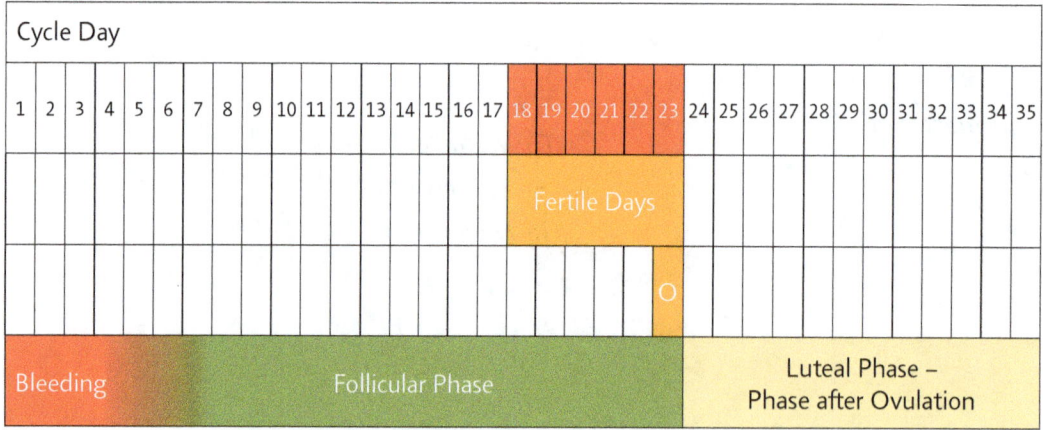

O = Ovulation

42 Day Cycle with Late Ovulation on Day 29

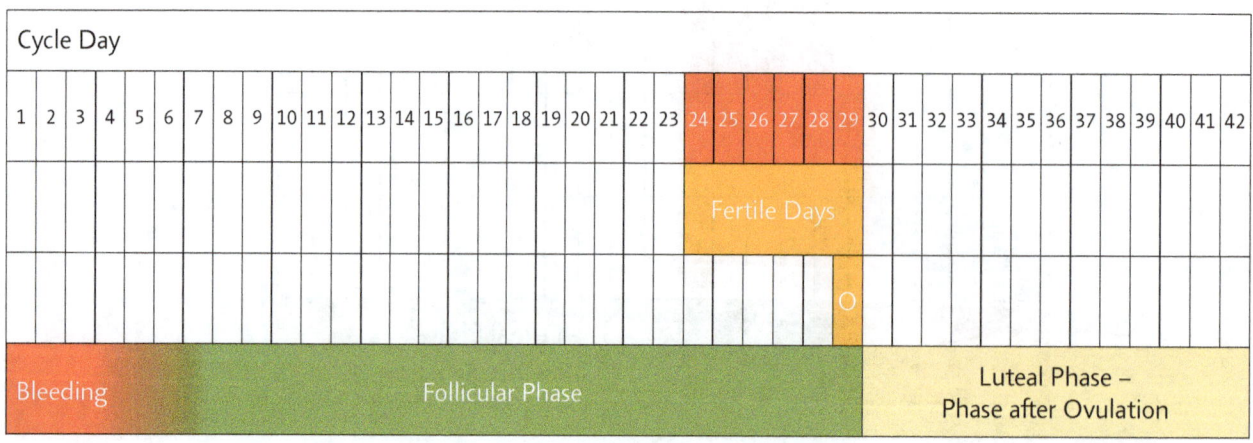

O = Ovulation

When Am I Fertile?

There are certain circumstances that a woman could become pregnant during her period: if a cycle is short and ovulation occurs early, or if she has mistaken an ovulation bleed for her period. Only women who observe their cycle are able to recognize this.

FACT
When women experience a long cycle which lasts, for example, eight weeks, some reckon that a "period has skipped" between two cycles. This is not the case; only one cycle has taken place. The egg ripening was extended over several weeks, and ovulation took place about two weeks before the next period.

FACT
The cervical mucus is the best and simplest sign of fertility! Whoever sees or feels the Magic Potion knows that it is possible for the sperm to survive and wait for ovulation! Good if you wish to have children, but not good if a pregnancy is not intended!

The Myth about the Second Ovulation
Again and again, it is claimed that ovulation occurs twice or more during one cycle. This is a persistent rumor because women report getting pregnant just shortly before their period, around day 28 of the cycle. They have been taught that ovulation takes place on day 14 and now have to assume that the ovulation which led to the pregnancy was a second, extra ovulation. In reality everything went according to plan, the first and only ovulation just happened to take place later this time. When twins or triplets occur, then ovulation does take place several times, but never more than six hours between each ovulation and only during the one fertile window.

9 The Cycle Show Put to the Test
Various Types of Cycles and their Causes

The female body is incredibly strong and adaptable; therefore it is not surprising that women have the responsibility of pregnancy and childbirth. A woman is not a machine, functioning constantly and consistently on demand; it is part of her passionate nature to experience the ups and downs of life with great intensity. She doesn't remain completely unaffected by these experiences but acts, thinks, and feels with her heart and mind, body, and spirit.

Whether her cycle is smooth or bumpy, long or short, the way it takes place in her body is a good indicator of her well-being. "Show me your cycle and I'll tell you how you're feeling!" Unfortunately, the body's signals and reactions are quite often misunderstood.

Attention! Attention! Warning Signals from the Top

A young athlete is very unhappy because she has irregular periods. She thinks her body is not functioning correctly, when in fact the very opposite is true: her body is reacting perfectly. How is this so? Well, think about what happens if you accidentally touch something hot. You'd pull your hand back immediately because the pain penetrates your body, warning you of danger. Similarly, these "cycle disturbances" are also clever warning signals; they are the body's way of adapting to various situations in life.

Young girls can experience different stresses: family quarrels, a parent's divorce, worrying about school grades and exams, problems with friends, and the first experience of feeling "lovesick." Teenagers don't necessarily treat their bodies with respect. Loud music, all-night parties, smoking and alcohol, lack of sleep,

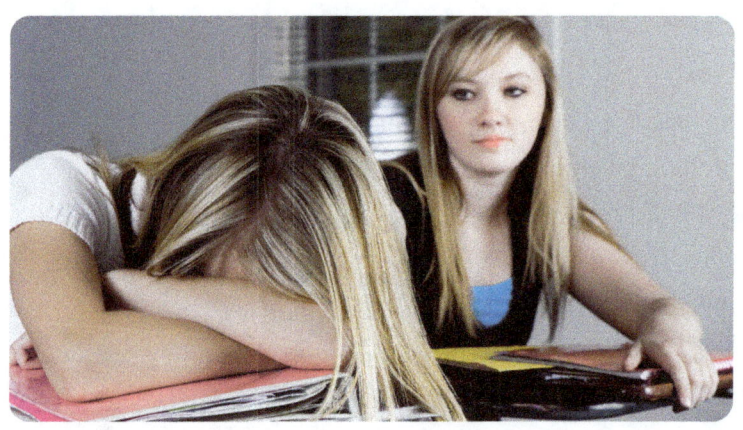

Teenagers can experience a variety of stresses, including family quarrels, a parent's divorce, worrying about school grades and exams, problems with friends and the first experience of feeling "lovesick."

and permanent tiredness are all current aspects of young modern lives.

It doesn't get much better in later years. Many women are exposed to the multiple stresses of juggling a career, relationship, family and household responsibilities. They seldom get time for themselves and little time to sleep.

Our bodies are not only subjected to unpleasant events. Unusual situations, such as traveling, changing environment, or taking a vacation, can also place a burden on the body. This all means STRESS. There are girls and women who are unaffected by these events, and their cycles continue to run smoothly; they are rock solid, with no reaction to external influences. However, this is not always the case. If everything gets too much for the body, then it provides itself with a break by shifting down a gear; sometimes it is even forced to take energy-saving measures. The cut backs are initially made where it hurts least, where there is luxury and the finer things in life; hence, the cycle events are always the first to be affected.

This results in cycle changes, often called "cycle disorders," can take on varying forms and often merge into one another.

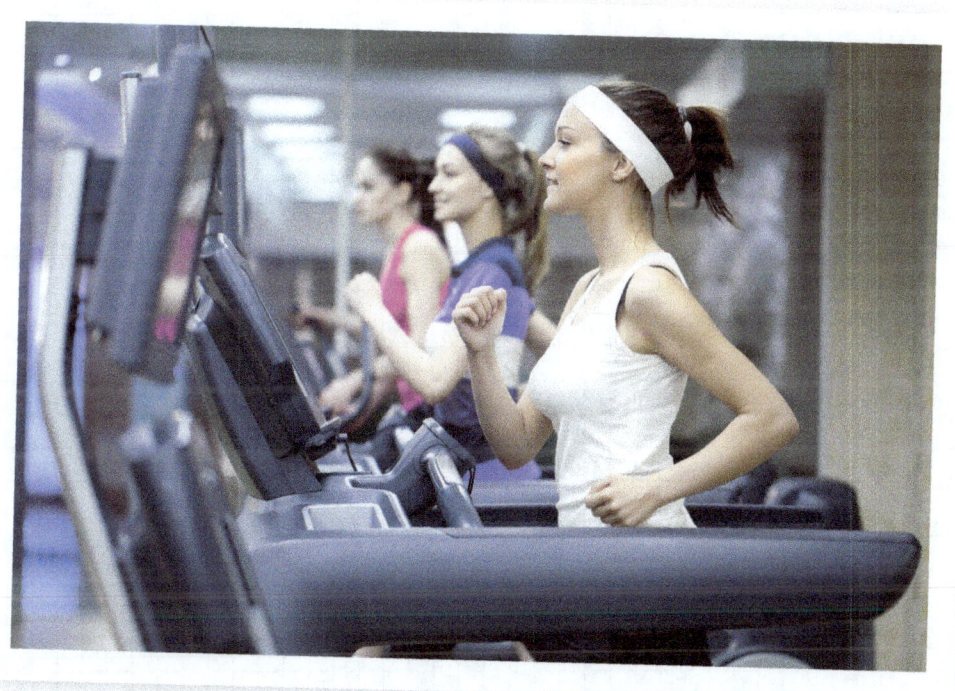

Various physical activities can put a strain on young women's bodies. If the boundaries are overstepped, this results in stress at the management level. Cycle disorders in this case are nothing more than warning signals.

Stress Type A: Delayed Ripening of the Egg

The normal cycle length ranges between 23 and 35 days. As already described, it is quite normal that women occasionally experience an unusually long cycle; however, it is more of a problem if the cycles are always longer than 35 days. In this case, the ripening of the egg is delayed to such an extent that ovulation may only take place four or five times a year. Doctors call this oligomenorrhea.

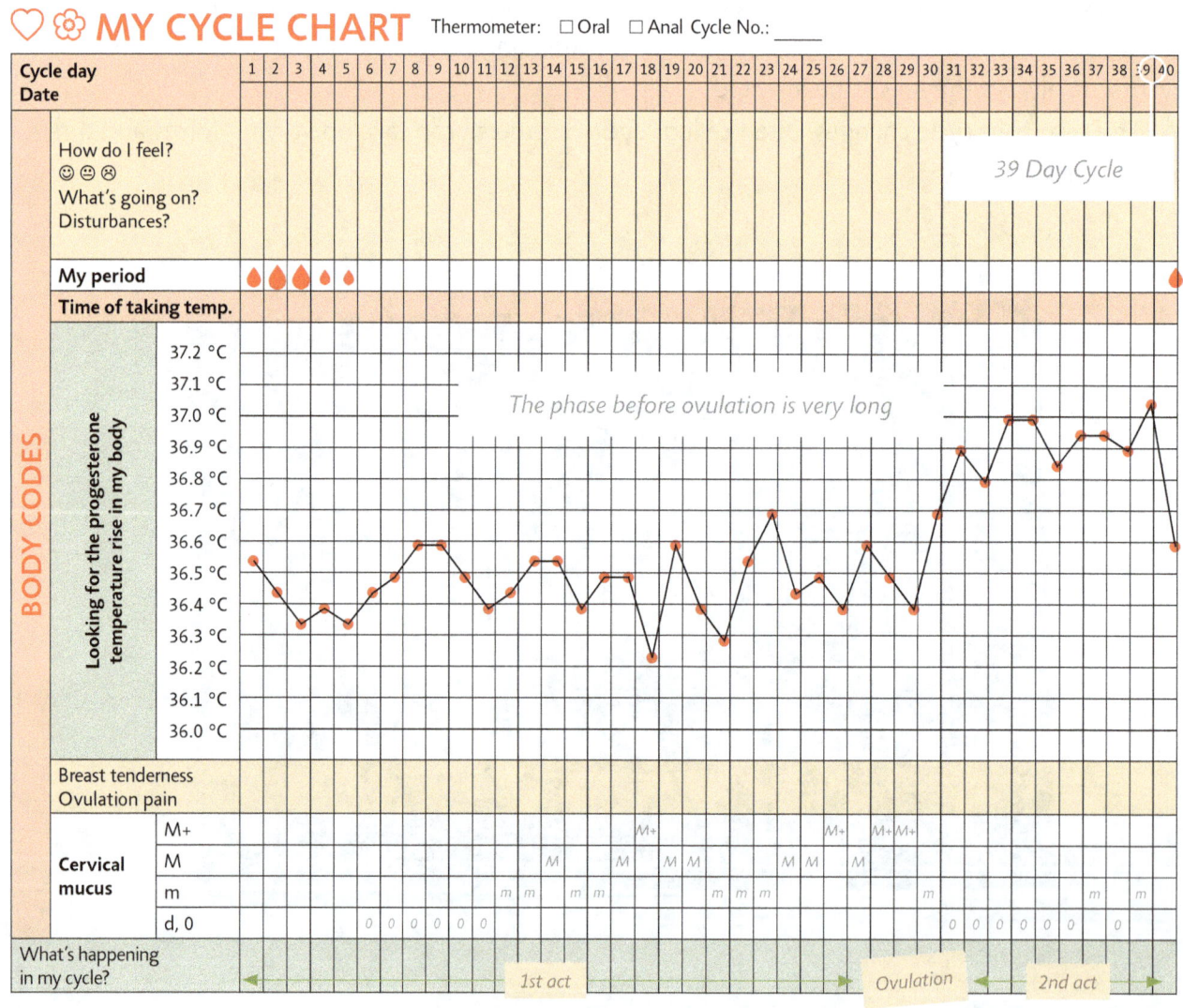

Cycle with delayed ovulation: it takes roughly 4 weeks until ovulation occurs.

Stress Type B: Cycle Without Ovulation

The egg requires great courage to take its adventurous leap, so thorough preparation is required. Everything must be finely tuned, to the very last detail, otherwise things can go wrong. The egg needs a great deal of external support from the Ovulation Helpers sent by the Control Center in the brain. Coordination problems can arise with the estrogens due to stress. Ovulation can only take

> **FACT**
>
> A cycle in which ovulation does not occur is called anovulatory. Due to the fact that there is no increase in temperature, it is also known as a monophasic cycle. Although there was no ovulation, and subsequently no second phase of the cycle, the woman does have her period because the estrogens have already built up the uterine lining in the first phase of the cycle.

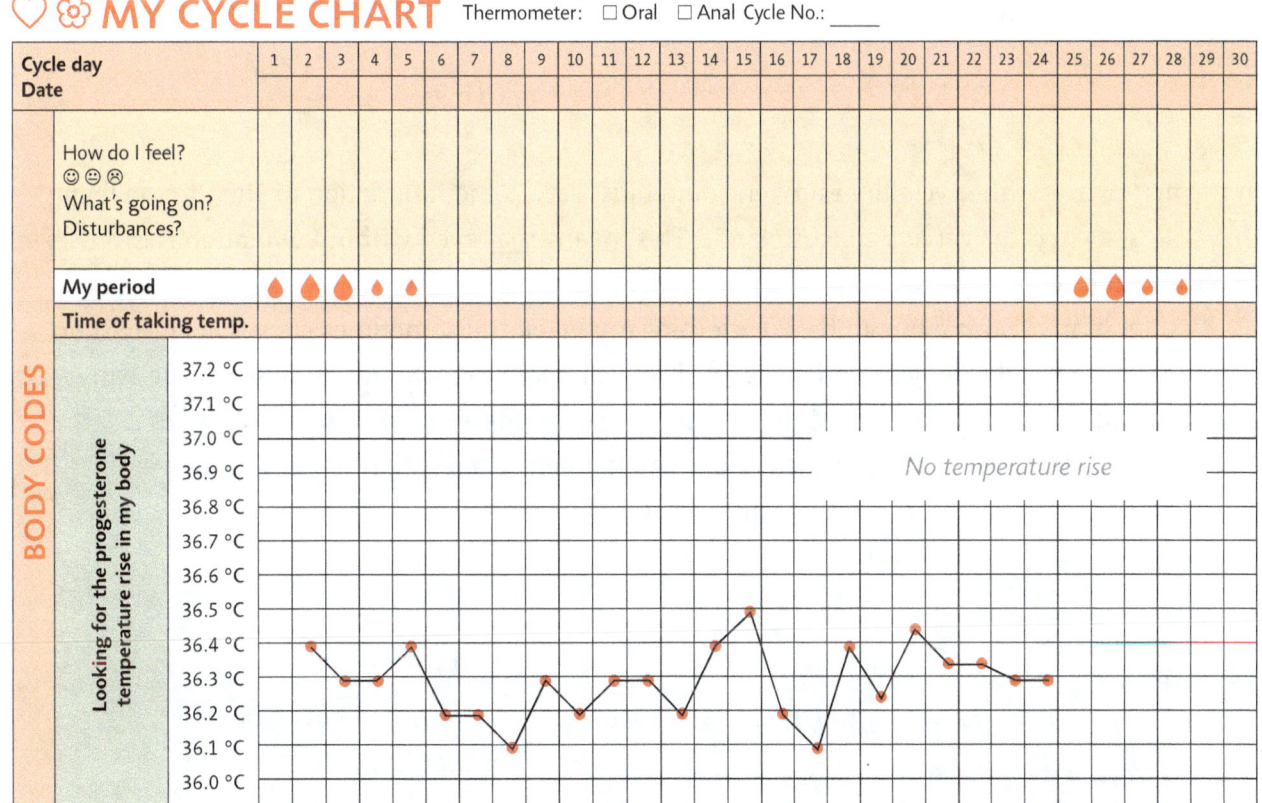

Example of a "monophasic cycle," in which ovulation does not take place and as a result the second phase of the cycle does not occur.

place when estrogen concentration is at a certain level in the blood for a certain length of time. If the estrogens weaken slightly, they fail to persuade the managers to release the luteinising hormone and ovulation doesn't occur. The egg remains in the ovary and slowly dissolves; the follicle shrinks and produces no further estrogens.

Without ovulation, no corpus luteum is formed, and no luxurious decoration of the uterine lining takes place; the second phase of the cycle is absent. The structural work set up by the estrogens, which was almost completed, is no longer needed. The period will start eventually, even without ovulation, but it is not a real period because it was not preceded by the luteal phase. It can't be possible to tell the difference when looking from the outside of the body, or can it?

> **How can you find out if ovulation took place?**
> With a thermometer and a few logical conclusions:
> Without ovulation
> - The corpus luteum cannot develop from the collapsed follicle.
> - The Progesterone Team are not produced.
> - The body temperature is unable to increase in the absence of progesterone.

What about the Cervical Mucus?

In the first phase of the cycle the estrogens didn't just set up the foundation of the uterine lining, they also activated the cervical mucus glands. This means that even without ovulation it is possible to observe the cervical mucus.

The duration of such a monophasic cycle can vary in length, sometimes it's suspiciously short but often it is normal in length, and looks just like a standard Cycle Show. Sometimes the whole thing can last six to twelve weeks. Without using a thermometer, no one would know that ovulation and the second phase of the cycle didn't happen. Interestingly, up until the age of 20, approximately every sixth cycle is still without ovulation.

> **FACT**
> The second phase of the cycle, also known as the luteal phase, usually lasts about 10 – 16 days. If it is shorter than 10 days, then it is referred to as a luteal insufficiency.

Stress Type C: Shortened Luteal Phase

The corpus luteum becomes active in the second phase of the cycle, when the Progesterone Team swarm out. It takes time to do a good job in preparing the uterine lining; at least ten days are needed (more usually 10 to 16 days), measured by the raised body temperature. At a particular age or in a certain life situation, the Service Center, the corpus luteum,

The luteal deficiency becomes a problem when a woman wants to have a child. Fertilization does actually occur in these cycles because the estrogens have provided the Magic Potion and the sperm were able to reach the egg, but a week later, when the embryo arrives in the uterus and hopes to find the Luxury Suites, the party is already breaking up. The Progesterone Team, whose job it was to take care of the new life, has already packed up and left and is no longer available to provide the necessary services. Even if menstruation has not yet begun, there is no support and the embryo must die.

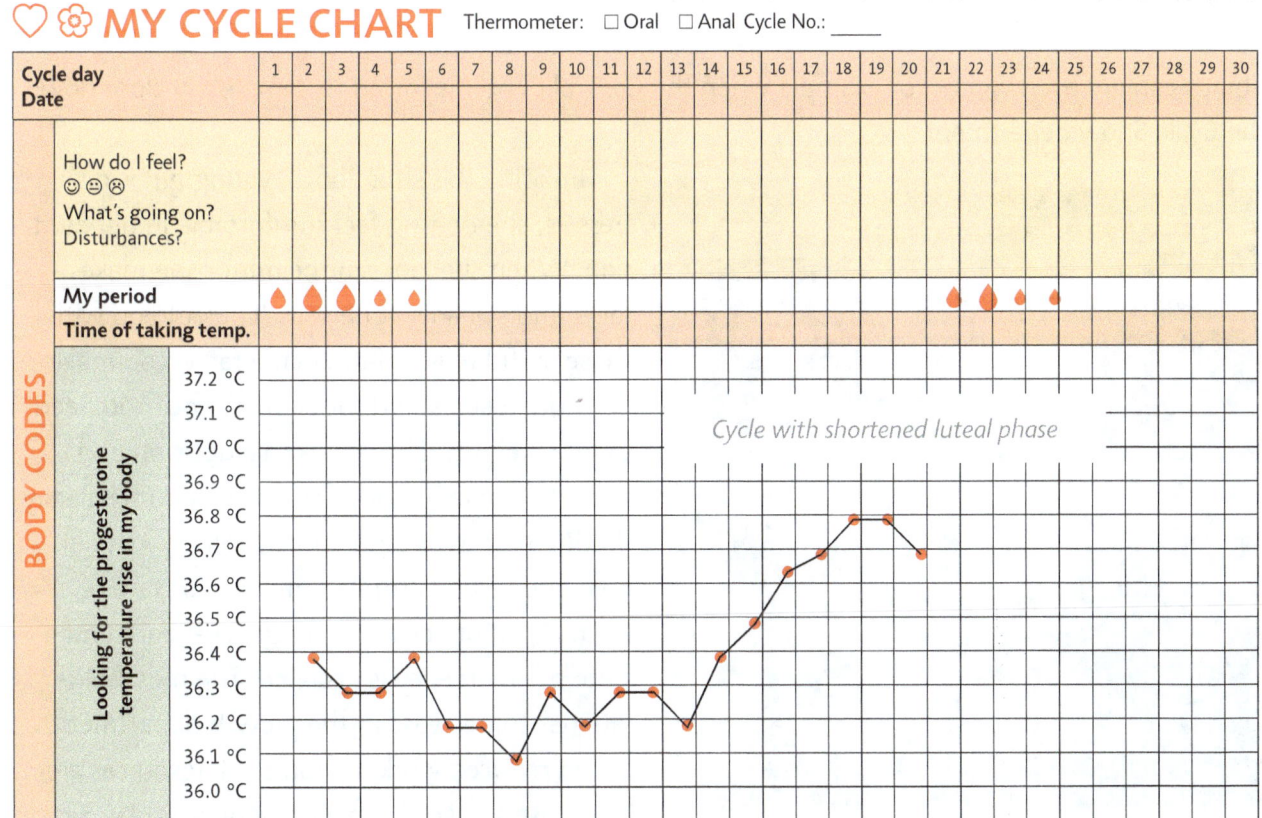

In this cycle the luteal phase only lasts one week.

may run out of steam too early. It is possible that there isn't enough progesterone available after nine, eight, seven, or sometimes even fewer days, so the uterine lining can no longer be maintained and is washed away with the period and the temperature drops.

Luteal deficiency is completely normal in girls and young women. This type of cycle is also frequently found during the menopause, after birth, during breast-feeding or after coming off the pill or other hormonal contraception. In addition to these exceptional situations, the many stresses which women are under can often lead to the second phase of the cycle being shortened.

> **FACT**
>
> *If a woman has not had a period for over three months, it's referred to as amenorrhea. Among other things the reasons for this can be extreme physical and mental strain due to eating disorders (anorexia, bulimia nervosa or obesity), competitive sports and also certain illnesses.*

Stress Type D: No More Periods

Things can get even worse, for example when the Control Center is forced to completely close down the Cycle Show department.

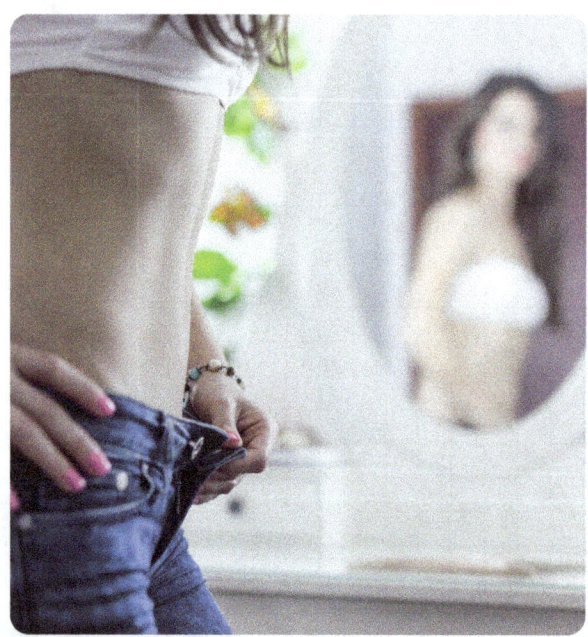

The cycle often reacts very sensitively to diets.

Imagine this situation. A young girl is distressed; she doesn't feel comfortable in her own skin. When she looks in the mirror she makes faces and screams at herself: "Look at you with those awful rolls of fat, what a fatty, you make me sick! I can't stand the sight of you! You need to lose weight!" She comes to a decision and starts to starve herself; drastically and mercilessly shedding pounds with an iron will against her own body. The Control Center is in a state of great agitation, crisis meetings take place and a state of emergency is declared. The metabolic rate has to decrease as the growth department are on reduced working hours. All resources are being used to keep the vital cardiovascular system going. At least budget cuts can be afforded here.

But then what happens to the Cycle Show division? What happens to the Messengers of Spring? Such luxuries can no longer be afforded in these hard times. They are told they are "not vital for life" and are dismissed. This is the end of the Cycle Show.

This has major consequences. If the FSH doesn't get to wake up the eggs, then that's the end for the estrogens in the body. The uterine lining will not be built up and there will be no more cervical mucus. No single egg will be chosen and ovulation will not take place. This means there will also be no progesterone and the uterine hotel remains unbuilt and unfurnished. There are no Luxury Suites to flow out of the body when no longer needed; the period never happens.

This amenorrhea is the most dramatic reaction of the body to a high level of stress. If a period doesn't occur for more than half a year, then it's possible that the body may not have enough estrogen at its command. We know estrogen is crucial for a woman's wellbeing; she cannot live healthily without these true friends, at least not long term. In the worst of cases this can do damage to the body, affecting the strength of her bones, which could lead to osteoporosis. The best thing would be to eliminate the actual cause of the amenorrhea as quickly as possible, but if this fails, it could be necessary in such cases to supply the body temporarily with estrogen substitutes.

Follicular phase (days 1–14)	Luteal phase (days 15–18)	*Shortened luteal phase "luteal insufficiency"*
Follicular phase (days 1–23)	Luteal phase (days 24–28)	*Prolonged follicular phase, shortened luteal phase*
Insufficient egg maturation – No ovulation (days 1–29)		*Monophasic cycle, anovulatory cycle*
(days 1–81 etc, no phases marked)		*"Amenorrhea" no period for more than three months*

Breakdown in Other Departments of the Control Center

Naturally not every serious disturbance in the cycle can be blamed on the stressful influences mentioned above. It may be that the Cycle Show department is unjustly affected due to bad administration in other departments of the Control Center.

The same disturbances may then also occur in the Cycle Show. In order to rule out a physical illness, it is advisable to recognize prolonged disturbances and consult a doctor.

The whole Control Center may be plunged into chaos if:
- The thyroid is under or overactive.
- The sugar metabolism has become imbalanced.
- Milk producing hormones are being activated, even when not breastfeeding.
- Too many male hormones are being produced due to a disruption of the hormonal metabolism (as with the PCO Syndrome).

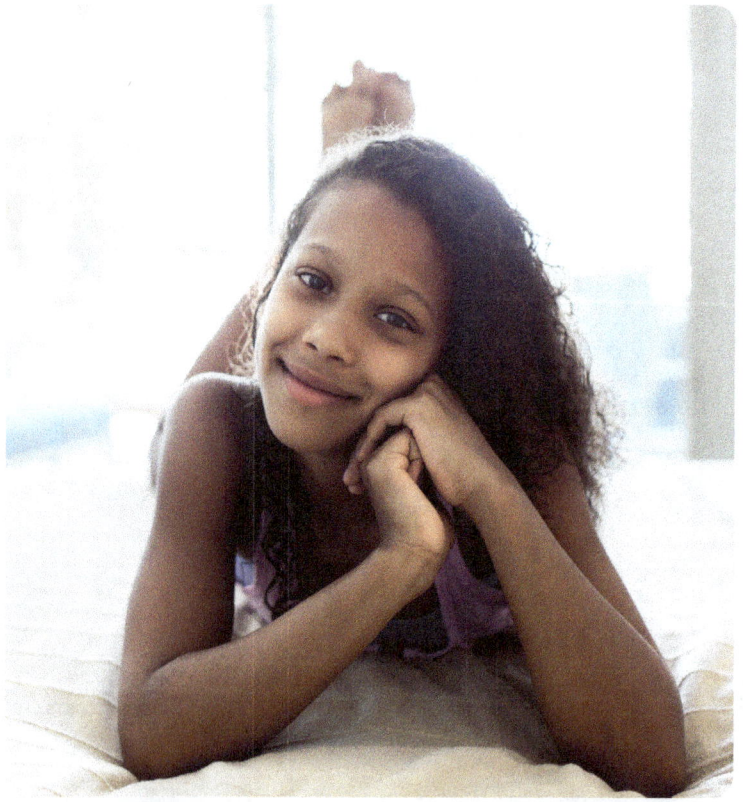

To feel comfortable in one's own body has a positive influence on the cycle.

Quickly and Smoothly: Thank You from the Control Center

Fortunately it's not only bad news that reaches the brain. If a girl feels comfortable in her own skin, this is like a declaration of love to the management. If she really looks forward to a vacation, a friend's visit or the many exciting things life offers, the "happiness hormones" swarm out around her body and can perform many miracles in the brain. In these perfect conditions, the eggs mature normally and ovulation takes place regularly. This is always a positive sign, a thank you from the management for the good teamwork.

10 The Effect of Different Contraceptive Methods on a Woman's Body

If the last two chapters were of interest to you, then this book may well have accompanied you for a number of years. Now you are a young woman, giving things a great deal of thought and dreaming of happiness, perhaps a boyfriend, and the possibility of falling in love. When your parents or caretakers try to discuss this subject with you, you can sense their worry about an unplanned pregnancy. Naturally, you don't want this to happen either. If you look for information, you'll find a lot of advise on how to best "protect" yourself against the "danger" of an unwanted pregnancy on the internet, publications, brochures, and schools.

Often the solution sounds quite simple: "Take the birth control pill and use a condom, and all is well!" However the simple solutions we all long for don't always exist, especially not in this situation. It's not simply a matter of whether to take the birth control pill, use a condom, or both; it is about something much more important. It concerns the body, mind, and emotions of two people. It concerns their health and well-being, closeness and tenderness, physical pleasure, and passion. It is a matter of trust, respect, and consideration; it's about love and fidelity. Furthermore, it's about the future and new life.

If we think of all the unintended pregnancies which continue to occur, despite the availability of information and free access to contraception, then it becomes clear that deciding to have sex, even nowadays, still includes the possibility of becoming pregnant. So how do we deal with it? In order to be able to make responsible decisions we need to be well informed, with accurate knowledge of the human body and how it works.

This book attempts to provide important and easy to understand information. It details the effects that contraceptive methods have on a woman's body and how it affects her fertility cycle. This vital information is not generally found on the internet or in sex education books and pamphlets, which are widely available. It can only be properly understood if you have a good working knowledge of the menstrual cycle, as presented in the previous chapters. Based on this knowledge you can form your own opinion, weigh up the possible advantages and disadvantages, and deal with your body, sexuality and emotions in a responsible way.

The Equation of Life is No Longer Valid

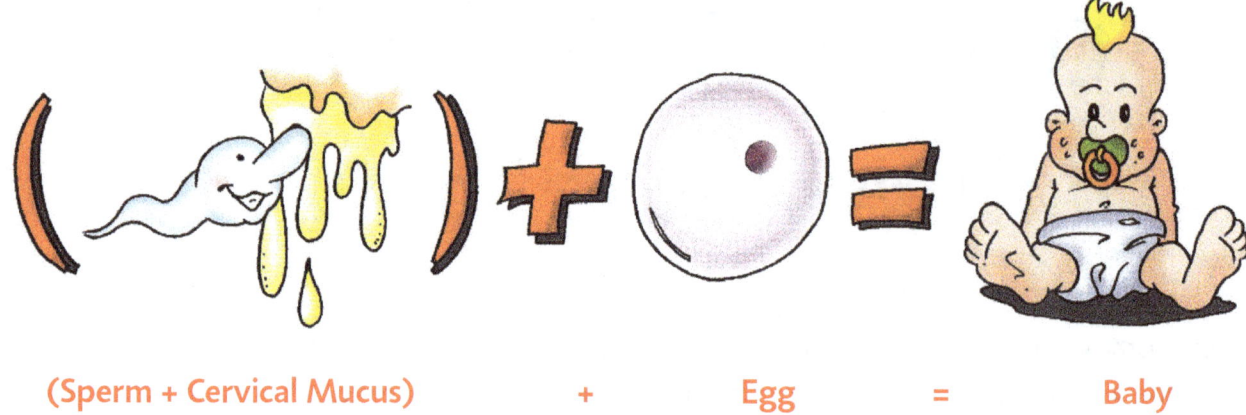

(Sperm + Cervical Mucus) + Egg = Baby

If sperm are present in the cervical mucus during the fertile period and manage to fuse with the egg, then a new human being is created. The Equation of Life becomes a reality.

Most methods of contraception work in such a way that one part of this equation is removed. If the sperm are removed from the equation, then it is easy on the woman's body and it doesn't influence her fertility cycle. This is the case when a condom, diaphram, cervical cap, male sterilization, or the unreliable principle behind using withdrawal is used.

However, if the production of the cervical mucus, the ripening of the egg, or ovulation is prevented, this often means more interference with the fertility cycle and the bodily processes. When sperm and egg have already fused together and the Equation of Life has become a reality, the further development of the embryo could be stopped.

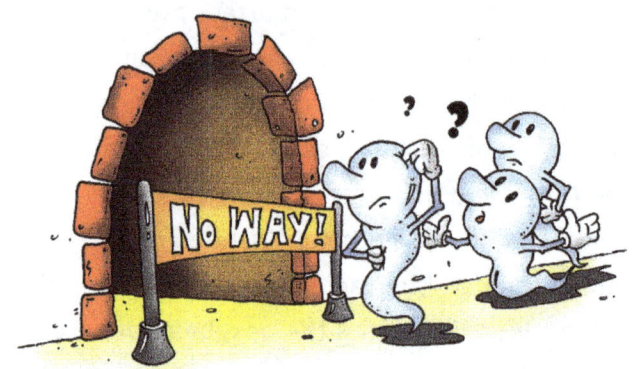

Combined Oral Contraception (COC/Birth Control Pill) – The Effect on the Cycle Show

If you ask most people how the birth control pill actually works, they will tell you that it "prevents ovulation" or "imitates pregnancy." There is some truth in these answers; however, neither is completely correct.

The Pill Cycle – Artificially Produced Shutdown Agreement Right from the Start

The birth control pill functions in such a way that simultaneously both an estrogen and a progesterone substitute are supplied. These highly effective artificial hormone substitutes have a certain similarity to the Estrogen Friends produced by the follicle and the Progesterone Team produced by the corpus luteum. These substances are transported through the bloodstream to the brain. When a woman starts to take the birth control pill, from the very first day, an artificial progesterone substitute (= progestogen) enters the body, but at a completely different point in the natural cycle. The Progesterone Team normally starts their work following ovulation, in the second phase of the cycle, so the Control Center is unable to recognize this deception and presumes ovulation has already taken place. The Shutdown Agreement is immediately put in place, just like in the natural cycle, and prevents the Messengers of Spring from being sent to the ovaries and waking up the eggs. Therefore, no ovulation takes place. If this Shutdown Agreement is in effect from the very first day of use, then, as a result, the entire natural cycle is stopped.

Although there are various types of birth control pills, they are all based on the same principle. By means of the progesterone substitute (= progestogen), the hypothalamus and the pituitary gland are misled, therefore, the Control Center in the brain fails to give the stage directions. But what are the consequences of this? The woman has no natural cycle anymore; the estrogen substitutes don't play any great role in the action, but are supplied so that she doesn't suffer from the side effects of a lack of estrogen.

> **FACT**
> *Some types of the birth control pill, like the multiphasic birth control pill, try to simulate the natural course of the cycle. They contain a little amount of estrogen substitute in the beginning, a larger amount in the middle; and then a smaller amount in the third phase. However, because of the Shutdown Agreement, the natural fertility cycle has already ended.*

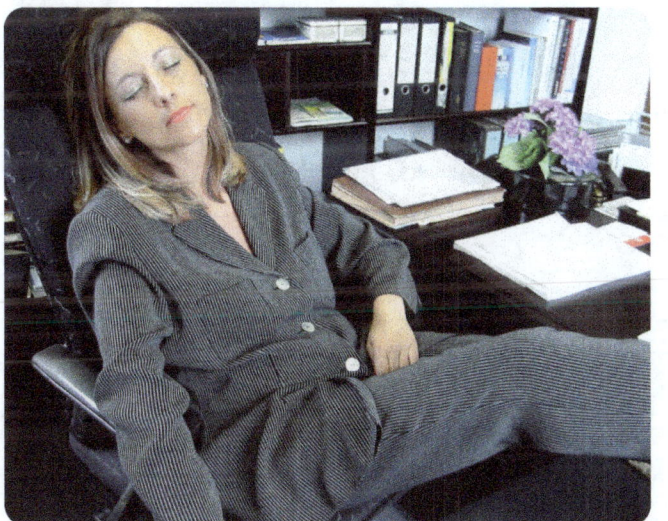

Ovaries Stop Working

The ovaries stop working and the eggs remain in hibernation. The naturally produced estrogens are no longer swarming around the woman's body and looking after her wellbeing.

Effect on the Uterine Lining

Of course the birth control pill hormones also turn up in the uterine lining, but not like in a normal cycle when one hormone comes after the other. In a normal cycle, first the estrogen builds up the mucous membrane, and then the progesterone looks after the interior decoration. With the birth

> Progesterone is the term for the naturally produced progesterone. Progestogen is the collective term for all artificially produced substitutes.

control pill, both hormone substitutes appear at the same time, and they keep getting in each other's way. While the estrogen substitute is trying to build the foundations, the progestogen is already starting the interior decorating and bringing in the furnishings. The result is far from harmonious; the

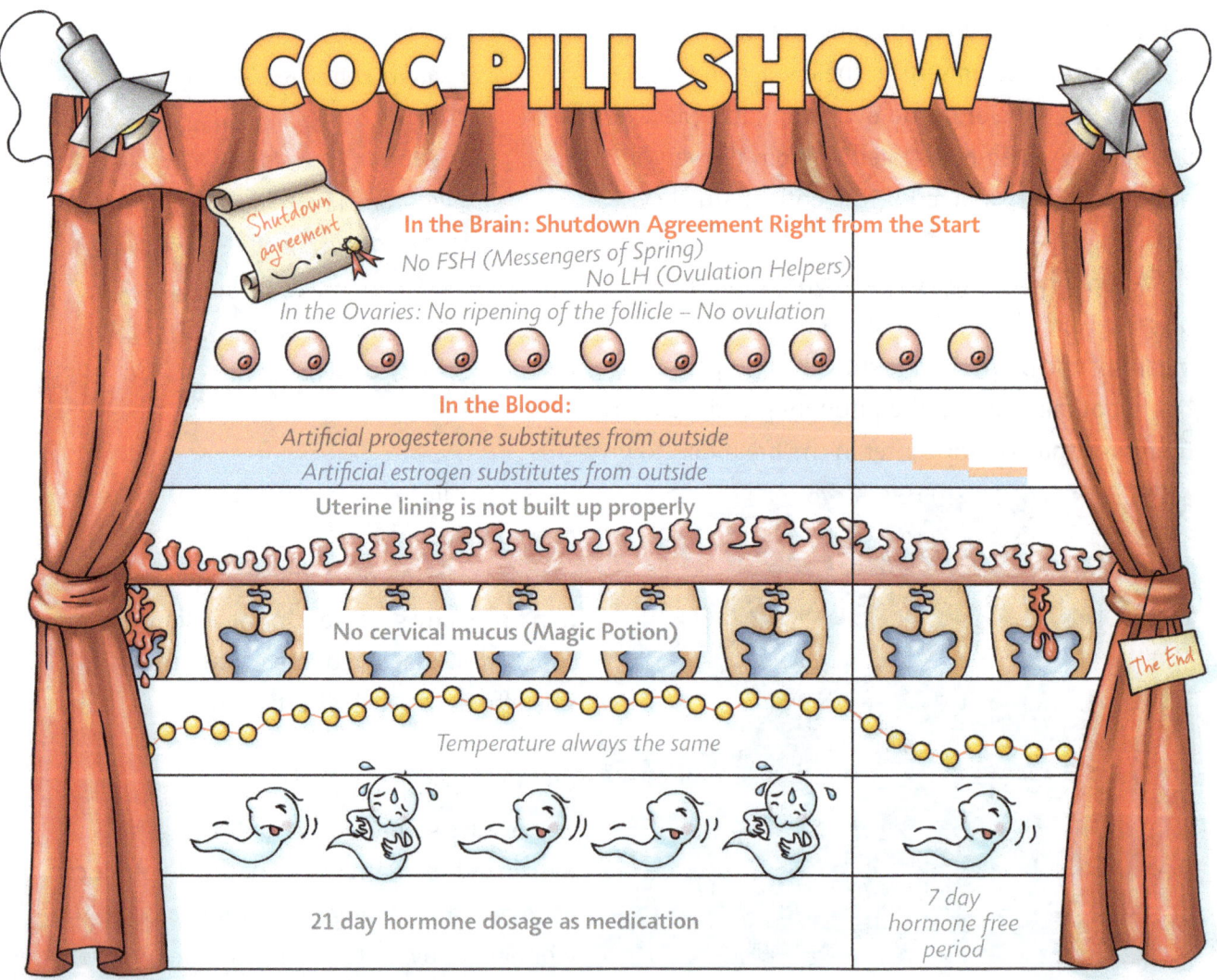

walls are unstable and lopsided, the ceilings are far too low and the inner furnishings remain sparse. Far from being luxurious, the hotel is pretty uninhabitable! Especially in the first months of taking the birth control pill, it is possible that the amount of estrogen substitute is not high enough so that nothing can be built up and the period doesn't happen.

Intermenstrual bleeding can occur when the concentrations of hormones are too low. This has nothing to do with a period but is merely a reaction of the uterine lining to the low hormone level. In these cases, doctors speak in terms of a lack of "cycle control," meaning there can be other bleeds that occur in between the withdrawal bleed brought on by the seven day break in taking the birth control pill.

Many women attach great importance to having a period every four weeks, so they think that something is wrong with "their cycle" when intermenstrual bleeding occurs while taking the birth control pill. They should, of course, be aware that Chlamydia can cause intermenstrual bleeding and be tested to exclude infections or problems with the cervix. Above all, they need to know that on the birth control pill, their cycle is artificial, and the bleed is only created by the drop in the hormone substitutes.

The Effect of the Birth Control Pill on the Cervical Glands

In the natural cycle, following ovulation, when the progesterone is at work, sperm die within a very short time in the vagina. They find themselves stranded in an acidic environment with no Magic Potion to protect them and a thick plug of mucus blocks the cervix preventing them from progressing. The birth control pill imitates these natural events. Instead of what is happening in every second phase of the natural fertility cycle, the progesterone substitute starts with the first birth control pill and is active throughout. The cervical mucus has dried up, the cervix remains closed, and no changes can be observed. The discharge that some women see when taking the birth control pill usually has nothing to do with the Magic Potion.

FACT
The main effect of the birth control pill is to stop the Control Center in the brain from working. There is no natural cycle anymore.

FACT
The birth control pill doesn't simulate pregnancy, just the second phase of the cycle!

At Times Constantly Raised: The Body Temperature

Even the temperature regulation center in the brain is taken in by the deception. Since the progestogen is already in the body from the first day of taking the birth control pill, the temperature stays at the same level all the way through the cycle. Some pharmaceutical formulations cause the temperature to rise immediately and to remain at this increased level the whole time the birth control pill is being taken. Since there is no natural fertility cycle, it is not possible to make a judgement based on the body temperature.

The End of the Story – Hormone Substitute Withdrawal Bleeding

In a natural cycle, the menstrual bleeding is triggered by the withdrawal of the corpus luteum as soon as it realizes no guest has arrived. The hormone concentration drops so that the uterine lining can no longer be maintained and is washed out of the body with the blood during the period.

This process is somewhat different on the birth control pill. The concentration of the hormone substitutes does in fact decrease; however, this is not due to the decision of the corpus luteum to abandon the job. Rather, it is because the pill package has come to an end after 21 days or that the remaining tablets to be taken do not contain hormone substitutes. As a result, even the sparse foundations which were built up by the birth control pill hormone substitutes in the uterus cannot be maintained any longer and bleeding begins. This is a hormone substitute withdrawal bleed. Since the building quality was rather substandard, the tidy up work passes quickly and easily. The birth control pill bleed is usually shorter, lighter, and less painful.

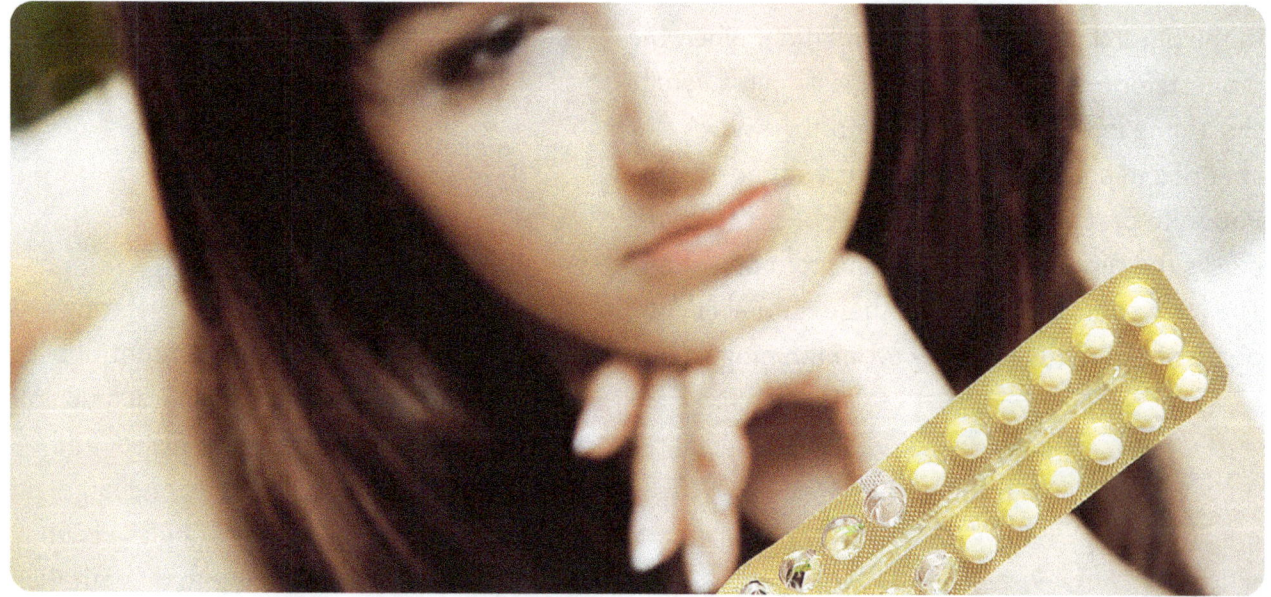

The birth control pill is a highly effective pharmaceutical formulation.

Phased Effect, Depending on the Concentration of the Hormonal Substitutes

The Natural "Fighting Spirit" of the Cycle Asserts Itself

So how come:
- Women sometimes observe clear cervical mucus?
- It is not uncommon for the doctor to discover growing follicles when doing ultrasound check-ups, occasionally even one that is mature and preparing for ovulation?
- The contraception can no longer be effective if two birth control pills are missed?
- Sometimes pregnancy occurs despite taking the birth control pill conscientiously?

The answer is:
In all of these cases the amount of hormone substitutes was just not high enough to completely suppress the "fighting spirit" of the natural cycle. There are a number of reasons for this.

What has been described up to now is what's known as the birth control pill's normal mode of action. The hormonal substitutes in the birth control pill stop the Control Center in the brain from working and generate a blockade at various levels; the ovaries remain in hibernation, the cervix is sealed up, and the uterine lining made uninhabitable. It is quite understandable why the birth control pill is considered a very effective method of contraception.

Reduced Dose of Estrogen Substitute

Over the years the concentrations of the hormonal substitutes have been reduced. When The birth control pill came onto the market in the 1960's, the amount of estrogen substitute the woman's body had to cope with was more than twice as high as today. These large doses often led to serious side effects. Since then, attempts have continually been made to lower the amount of the estrogen substitutes. However, there are certain disadvantages arising from this; one being the intermenstrual bleeding already mentioned.

Every Woman Reacts Differently

The main reason for the different effects is that for each woman, the amount of both hormone substitutes that reach the places of action can vary, and each body deals with it differently. For example, body weight can play a role; the dose could be too high for a woman who is slim, while for a woman with a higher proportion of body fat, it may not be enough to completely block the Control Center in the brain.

Other factors can have an even greater influence on whether the birth control pill manages to shut down the natural cycle; such as the speed at which the birth control pill hormone substitutes can be broken down in the liver and the amount of protein in the blood binding with the hormones and making them inactive. A woman's diet can also interfere with the shutdown efficiency, as can how good she is at remembering to take her birth control pill regularly, which ensures a consistent hormone level in the blood. So while for some women there will be a total blockade in the brain of all cycle events, for others the effect of the birth control pill can vary.

The Shutdown Agreement No Longer Maintained

What happens when the concentration of progestogen in the brain is no longer sufficient to maintain the Shutdown Agreement? A problem arises for the birth control pill hormone substitutes because the Messengers of Spring in the brain are extremely enthusiastic and are always ready to get going. If the guard is let down for a very short time (e.g. the birth control pill is forgotten twice at the beginning of the cycle), then the FSH can no longer be restrained. The barriers are torn down and the Messengers of Spring storm off in the direction of the ovaries to do their job of waking up the eggs. This causes the growing follicles to produce different amounts of the body's natural estrogen, which can vary from one woman to the next.

Naturally Produced Estrogens Assert Themselves

It is possible that the naturally produced estrogen travels to the Leisure Center at the cervix and opens it. Magic Potion is on the menu once again, much to the delight of any sperm that may arrive! Now a woman can potentially observe stretchy, clear cervical mucus even when on the birth control pill.

Ovulation While on the Birth Control Pill

Whether a follicle will now be selected in the ovary is based on the concentration of the Messengers of Spring present, and how long they are allowed to function without interference. Even if a "Queen Egg" is chosen and develops sufficiently to ovulate, the amount of estrogen is usually insufficient to send the Ovulation Helpers into action. This means that in most cases ovulation never happens and the natural cycle events are stopped at this point. However, sometimes enough estrogen is available to motivate the pituitary gland to produce sufficient LH, in which case the woman ovulates while on the birth control pill.

Pregnant Despite the Birth Control Pill

It cannot be completely ruled out that sperm might have made their way through the available cervical mucus and managed to spend time on the Stage of Life. Fertilization is possible and the

Equation of Life can become a reality. We don't know enough about it yet, but it could be possible that the natural hormones in the body allow the uterine lining to prepare for implantation, despite the inhibiting action of the hormone substitutes. When women credibly claim that they have taken the birth control pill according to the instructions (without disturbances like diarrhea, vomiting, or certain medications) and have still become pregnant, then one can conclude that in these cases the embryo's will to live was very strong. It battled its way, against all odds, into the uterus and successfully settled down there.

> **FACT**
> *No contraceptive method is 100% reliable. The possibility of creating new life through sexual intercourse should always be kept in mind.*

Positive Effects of Natural Hormones on all Functions and Organs in a Woman's Body

The natural estrogens and progesterone don't just have an effect on the organs on the Stage of Life. The estrogens in particular are responsible for female identity, a fact which is not widely considered.

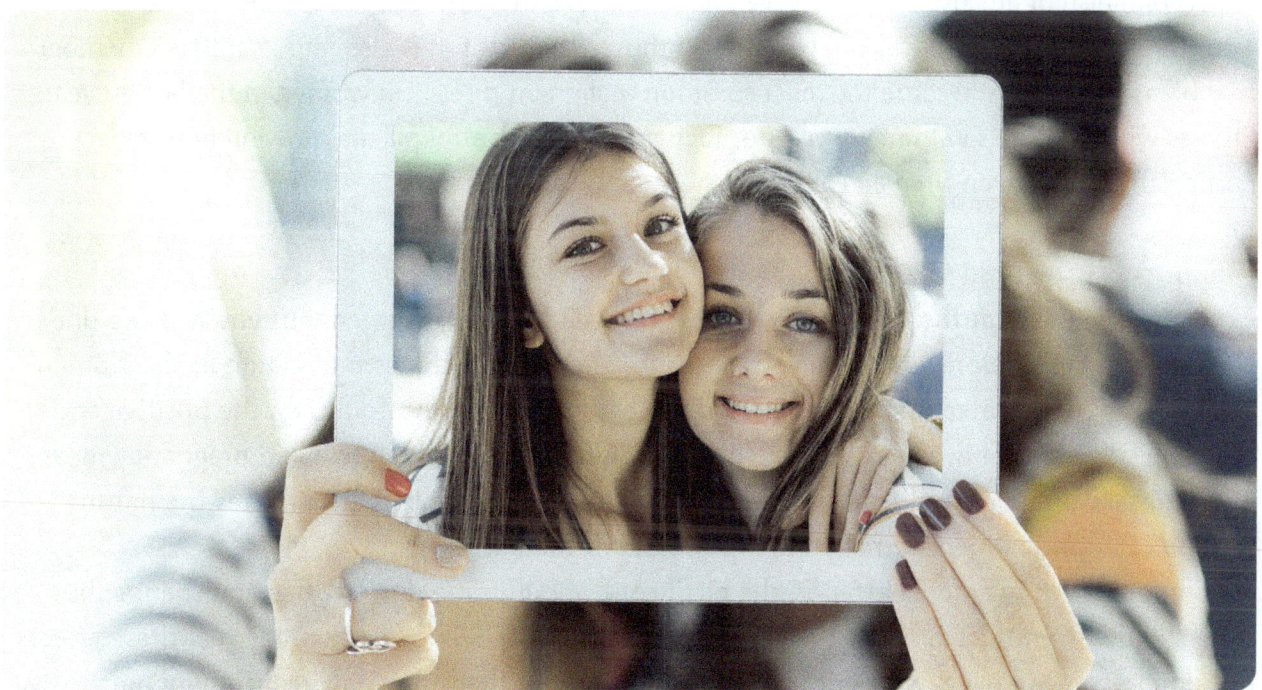

Natural estrogens are a woman's best friends and take care of her wellbeing.

Some women only realize what good friends they are when they experience some side effects due to the lower levels in menopause.

Most women don't know that their natural sex hormones influence virtually every cell and all of the functions and organs in their bodies.

> Natural estrogens and/or progesterone:
> - Build and repair a woman's bones and protect her against rapid bone loss.
> - Keep her skin and mucous membranes moist.
> - Make her hair shiny.
> - Decrease urinary infections.
> - Protect her heart and blood vessels, so she will have a significantly lower risk of strokes and heart attacks than men until menopause.
> - Have a positive influence on mood and mental state.

Natural Estrogens Replaced

So what changes when women take the birth control pill? First, the natural hormones are replaced by artificial substitutes. Some effects remain the same or are similar, but some of the protective effects diminish or are lost completely. Women who take the birth control pill are less protected from thrombosis, heart attack, and stroke than those who don't. It is also important to remember that breast cancer has become the most common malignant disease in women in the last 40 years. Studies which link this with many years of taking the birth control pill are growing in number, particularly when taken from an early age.

Making an Informed Choice

Experience shows that the birth control pill works well for many women, but you need to understand all the facts before you make your decision. The pill's mechanism of action in the woman's body is very complicated and in many respects not clarified. Many studies on the positive and negative side effects have been published. Taking the birth contol pill to avoid pregnancy means a daily intake of a highly effective pharmaceutical formulation, which deactivates the natural fertility cycle and influences many other processes in the body.

Some women may feel better on the birth control pill, some don't notice any change, but others know from the start that they "just don't feel right." Some women may feel these effects but don't associate them with hormonal contraception. Often they only realize how much better they feel when they stop taking it.

At different times in your life, different things will be important for you. It's up to you to weigh all of this from a position of knowledge.

Side Effects Become the Principal Effect

Painful Bleeding

Every woman is affected differently by her period; some have no problems and some suffer considerably. Young girls and women who suffer from heavy bleeding or menstrual cramps are very pleased that the bleed on the birth control pill is frequently shorter, lighter and less painful. This is because the uterine lining does not become so thick, so there is less to flow away. The pain relief is a positive side effect of the pill, but the principal effect is the deactivation of the natural cycle. So it is very important to consider whether the birth control pill is the right solution for you and your first choice when dealing with menstrual cramps.

In Order to "Control the Cycle"

Some girls and young women find it annoying when their period takes them by surprise and they are not prepared for it. They think that only a regular cycle is a healthy one and visit their doctor, who may prescribe the birth control pill for "cycle control." The pill-induced "regular cycle," however, is not her natural cycle; it has been replaced by the 28-day rhythm of the birth control pill. If she comes off the pill again, she will experience her own natural cycle as irregularly as before, and even more patience is required until everything "runs smoothly."

It is fascinating to discover the Cycle Show in your body, experience what is being performed, and understand why the show sometimes takes a break or lasts a little longer or shorter than expected.

> ### Coming off the COC Pill – Return of Fertility
> Half of the women who discontinue the birth control pill revert to their natural cycle within one to three cycles; the other half can expect disturbances in their fertility for up to a year. The Cycle Show is being rehearsed again and this requires being patient with the body.
> - Sometimes it takes weeks for ovulation to recur (prolonged follicular phase).
> - Sometimes the egg doesn't even make it this far (monophasic cycle).
> - Long after stopping the COC pill, the corpus luteum runs out of steam too early so the uterine lining cannot be sufficiently prepared (luteal deficiency).

Acne and Oily Skin

At puberty, some girls suffer greatly from acne and oily skin. Not only do the female hormones (estrogen and progesterone) enter the scene at this time, but also higher amounts of the male sexual hormones (androgens) appear with their leader: testosterone. They take up their positions, including the skin's sebaceous glands, and cause them to increase production. Being young, active, wild, and inexperienced, they frequently overshoot the mark causing an overproduction!

The progestogen contained in certain birth control pills is formed in a way that the sebaceous glands mistake it for the male sexual hormone and allow it to take up position at the command post. However, as it remains inactive, the secretion from the sebaceous glands decreases and the acne improves. This side effect of some birth control pills is now used as therapy for acne, but only you can decide if this benefit is worth deactivating your natural cycle.

Progestogen—Only Contraceptive Methods

Over the years much thought has been given to how hormonal contraceptive methods can be made with reduced side effects. The estrogens in particular have fallen into disrepute, and if listening to public debate, you could believe that estrogen was a danger to women's health, causing serious side effects such as thrombosis, stroke, and heart attack. The fact is that these side effects do not normally occur due to natural estrogen, but are triggered by the artificial estrogen substitute. To avoid

---

The Birth Control Pill in a Different Form: Vaginal Ring and Hormone Patch

The traditional COC pill is swallowed in tablet form. It travels to the intestine and then to the liver, where part of the hormone substitute is broken down without ever taking effect. Women who find taking a daily COC pill difficult, other ways have been devised to take the contraception. Instead of taking an oral tablet, the combined synthetic substitutes can be inserted into the vagina in the form of a vaginal ring or attached to the skin as a hormone patch. The respective estrogen and progesterone substitutes are released directly into the blood via the mucus membrane in the case of the vaginal ring or through the skin with the hormone patch. This method avoids the waste of hormone subsitutes in the liver, but apart from that they differ little from the COC pill in their effect and side effects.

these serious side effects, progestogen-only contraceptive methods have appeared on the market. They contain only a progestogen and no estrogen substitute and basically operate like the birth control pill. Once a sufficiently high quantity of progestogen is available in the blood, it reaches the brain and implements the Shutdown Agreement. This depresses the ripening of the follicle and its production of natural estrogen, but the estrogens (which are at least partly replaced when on the pill by the administration of estrogen substitutes) are missing here, and this has its consequences.

PROGESTOGEN-ONLY CONTRACEPTIVE METHODS

SYSTEMIC Effects
Via the Brain (hypothalamus and pituitary gland)
Prevention of Natural Cycle on Various Levels:

- "Shutdown Agreement" (negative feedback mechanism).
- Egg maturation.
- Ovulation.
- Formation of the corpus luteum.
- Production of body's natural hormones (estrogens and progesterone).

LOCAL Effects on:

- Cervical mucus.
- Uterine lining.

Progestogen-only Contraceptive Methods:

- Progestogen-only pill (POPs).
- Intrauterine System (IUS).
- The progestogen-only injection.
- Contraceptive implant.

The Desogestrel Containing POP and Other Progestogen-Only Pills

The desogestrel containing POP is also called the "mini pill" and should be taken from the first day of cycle without a break. It contains quite a high dose of progestogen and thus has a systemic effect on the female body with prevention of the natural cycle on various levels; little or no follicular growth, little or no natural estrogens, and suppression of ovulation.

> **Traditional POPs with Low Dose Progestogen**
> *The traditional POP's norethisterone (NET), and levonorgestrel (LNG) with low dose progestogen, are rarely used today. In return for the relatively small health burden which the traditional POP puts on the body, it is extremely important to take it at the same time each day. The hormone concentration is quite low, so that the effect is confined locally at the cervix and at the endometrium. Normally the natural course of the cycle should not be affected, but the reliability is lower compared with the desogestrel containing POP.*

The Intrauterine System (IUS)

The hormonal intrauterine System (IUS) is a small T-shaped plastic device, wrapped by a hormone reservoir. It is inserted through the cervix into the uterine cavity, and from there progestogen is continually released over a period of five years. The local effects are that the cervix is closed by a plug of mucus and the construction of the uterine lining is disrupted. Quite a significant proportion of women are not only locally but also systemically affected. Similar to the POP, the dose of hormones is high enough to stop the natural cycle.

> **FACT**
> **The New Low Dose Intrauterine System**
> The new, low dose hormonal intrauterine system remains in the uterus for three years. The plastic device and hormone reservoir is smaller, and is said to only have a local effect. The cervix is closed by a plug of mucus and the construction of the uterine lining is disrupted. Quite often it causes irregular bleeding.

Frequently No More Periods

The progestogen continually affects the uterine lining for years, and at first, irregular spotting occurs frequently. Often, the period becomes shorter and less heavy with time. When the uterine lining ceases to build up at all and the period stays away completely, it is referred to as a "uterine amenorrhea."

The Progestogen-only Injectable Contraceptives

The Progestogen-only injectable contraceptives act on the same principle. Depending on the preparation used, a depot of progestogen is injected subcutaneously or into the muscle every three months. The hormones are then released rather unevenly into the bloodstream from this reserve, a greater amount at the beginning and becoming less over the three months. The progestogen reaches the brain and implements the Shutdown Agreement, which depresses the ripening of the follicle, and leads to a decrease in the body's natural estrogen levels. These are similar to the low levels seen in the early phase of the menstrual cycle, and there is some evidence that use of progestogen-only injectable contraceptives can result in loss of bone mineral density (BMD). For this reason, young women who have not reached bone maturity (approximately at age 18) should seriously consider whether this method is suitable for them.

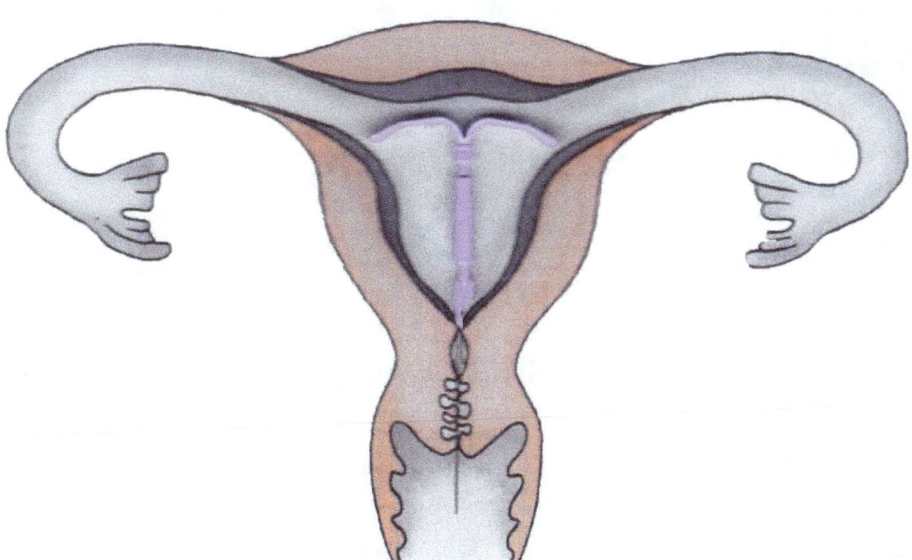

The intrauterine system releases progestogen over three or five years.

Contraceptive Implant

The contraceptive implant also has a systemic impact on a woman's body. It is implanted under the skin and releases consistent amounts of progestogen into the bloodstream over a period of three years. As a result, the blockade of the natural cycle comes into force at various levels in the body. With the activation of the Shutdown Agreement (the body's negative feedback mechanism), further follicle ripening is stopped and the production of the body's natural estrogen is gradually diminished.

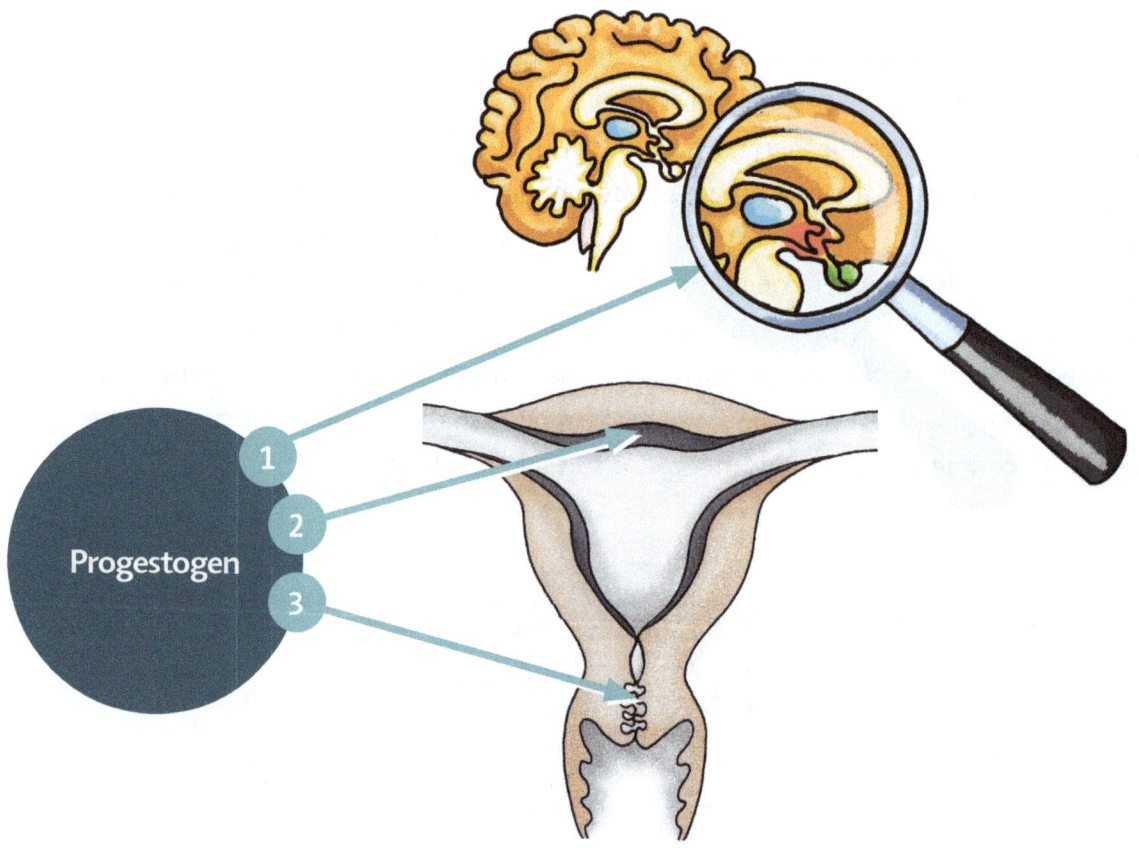

① Systemic effect at the brain: hypothalamus and pituitary gland

② Local effect at the uterine lining

③ Local effect at the cervix glands

This is how a progestogen works.

Uterine Lining – No Completion of the Interior without the Foundations

Once the small stick is implanted in the underside of the upper arm, the only thing that reaches the uterine lining for the next three years is the progestogen, whose job it is now to take care of the interior fittings like the natural progesterone did. However, no foundation will be built since there is no estrogen present, and, as there is no structural work, the completion of the interior is also impossible. Consequently, virtually no uterine lining will be built up, and no bleeding will occur. Some women are happy with it, but many complain about lengthy intermenstrual bleeding and spotting, and some have no bleeding at all (called "uterine amenorrhea"), which is thought to be caused by the constant presence of progestogen.

Caution! Where are the Estrogens?

These systemic progestogen-only contraceptive methods (desogestrel containing POP, contraceptive implants, the progestogen-only injectable, and maybe also the higher-dose intrauterine system) are highly effective, but one should consider the possible side effects. Some women who use these contraceptives complain of physical problems similar to menopause, such as hot flushes, profuse sweating, depression, dry mucous membranes, and a lack of sexual desire. In these cases, think about the possibility that the estrogen, the most important female hormone, is too low. Of course, there are differences in each woman's tolerance of these methods. Depending on body weight, metabolism, and many other physical and emotional factors, it ranges from "well tolerated" to "intolerable."

Young Girls Need Strong Bones!

The estrogen and progesterone produced in a natural cycle has a significant positive influence on a woman's health, especially her bones! It is well known that the natural cycle, with its fluctuating concentrations of estrogen, is the best prevention against osteoporosis in later life. A young woman whose bone growth is not fully completed should consider this when thinking about what contraception she might choose.

The Copper Intrauterine Device (Cu-IUD) – The Copper Coil

This non-hormonal method of contraception got its name because the first intrauterine devices actually looked like coils. It refers to a small plastic T-shaped device with a copper wire wound around it. The coil is inserted into the uterine cavity by a specially trained doctor or nurse. It remains there for about three to ten years, depending on the model, releasing copper ions into its surroundings.

> **FACT**
> Women who use the copper coil complain more often about painful, longer, and heavier periods. Five out of 100 coils are expelled.

Foreign Body in the Uterus – How Does the Copper Coil Work?

The Cycle Show is currently running. In the first cycle phase before ovulation, the estrogens are setting up the foundations in the uterus. Following ovulation, the Progesterone Team looks after the interior decoration. When a copper coil is inserted and lies in the uterine cavity, copper particles are continually released and strike the uterine lining like arrows. The work on the foundations and interior decoration is seriously disrupted; the walls are crooked, the plaster is crumbling, and the hotel is more like a ruin than a new building.

Initially the uterus fiercely defends itself against the coil and wants to get rid of it as quickly as possible. The muscles contract in its rebellion; the bleeding is heavier and lasts longer; and the abdominal cramps are much more severe. Sometimes the uterus succeeds in rejecting the coil, especially during the period when the tidying up work is already in progress.

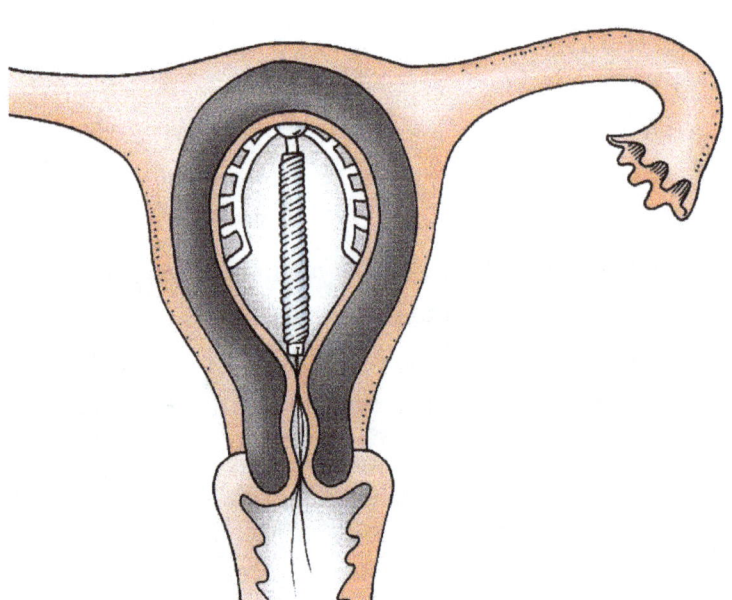

The position of a copper coil in the uterus.

A foreign body in the uterus causes the body's police force to go into action. White blood cells move in and try to encircle the coil in order to render it harmless, without any prospect of success.

Sperm in the Line of Fire

The sperm are also directly in the line of fire. Nothing good will await them if they leave the safety of the cervical mucus in the cervix and venture on further up. Many will either be hit by the copper particles, or harmed by the body's police force in the heat of the moment. Frequently, not a single sperm reaches the place of their dreams because they were destroyed along the way.

What if Fertilization Does Occur?

If however enough sperm manage to dodge the arrows and get as far as the fallopian tubes, then fertilization may occur. There is a further mode of action of the coil which will inhibit the embryo's journey. The fallopian tubes, which normally gently move the embryo through the narrow tunnel, are now caught up in the defensive measures against the copper particles, and as a result, are either moving too fast or too slow. For this reason, the embryo is sometimes pushed forward and arrives way too early in the uterus.

The Embryo Has No Chance of Survival

If the embryo reaches the uterus, then it has little hope of finding a quiet place there for the next nine months. The uterine lining has been rendered uninhabitable by the copper particles, and the body's defensive measures against the coil, and the embryo dies.

Ectopic or Tubal Pregnancy

Due to the disruption from the copper coil, the journey through the fallopian tubes may last too long. The embryo is now so big that it gets stuck in the fallopian tube and can't go any further, it decides to make the best of the situation and settle down on the spot and an ectopic pregnancy occurs. Unfortunately, the walls of the fallopian tube are completely unsuitable and much too thin to withstand the growing pressure for very long. Sooner or later cracks occur and bleeding arises, and if the problem has not yet been recognized then the situation can become life threatening for the mother if the fallopian tube bursts.

> **FACT**
>
> *The copper coil is offered to women as the most effective method of emergency contraption because it prevents implantation of the embryo.*

The Emergency Pill

The emergency pill is also called post coital contraception or the morning-after pill. It is used if there has been a "contraceptive slip up" or unprotected sex has taken place and pregnancy is not wanted.

There are two different types available at the moment, which differ in the mode of action. The first is 1.5mg of the progestogen levonorgestrel, which should be taken as soon as possible after unprotected sexual intercourse and can be taken up to three days after the contraceptive slip up. This corresponds to roughly five to ten times the amount of the progestogen dose in the birth control pill. The second preparation available contains the chemical substance ulipristal acetate, which is a progesterone receptor modulator and can be taken up to five days after unprotected intercourse.

Mode of Action of Progestogen and Progesterone Receptor Modulator

Both chemical substances act on the progesterone receptors. The progestogen levonorgestrel acts as a pure agonist, meaning that it tries to imitate the progesterone effects in the best possible way. Ulipristal acetate at certain times produces the opposite effect, however; before ovulation, it acts like progesterone (an agonist), but if ovulation and a subsequent fertilization had already taken place, then it acts as an antagonist. It displaces the progesterone from its receptors in the uterine lining, but without any activity. This could have consequences for any fertilized egg.

Women often do not know where they are in their cycle when taking the emergency contraception pill. Each type of pill will have a different mode of action depending on the phase of the cycle in which it is taken.

Situation 1: Ovulation Has Not Yet Taken Place

As noted in chapter 8, according to statistics, in every second cycle ovulation takes place after the 14th day, in every fifth cycle not until after the 20th day, and among younger girls and women it tends to be even later. So it must be assumed that in many cycles in which the emergency pill is taken, ovulation has not yet occurred. Before ovulation, both preparations have the same effect in that they occupy the progesterone receptors and try to mimic their normal activity. What does this mean? When they reach the brain via the blood, it mistakenly concludes that ovulation has already happened and the second cycle phase has begun. Immediately, the Shutdown Agreement is implemented, which interrupts the further maturation of the follicle and delays ovulation for a few days.

Situation 2: Ovulation is Currently Taking Place – Ovulation Helpers (LH) are Already Out and About

If unprotected intercourse happened around ovulation time and the emergency pill is taken only a few hours later, recent investigations suggest that levonorgestrel is not able to prevent ovulation and the following fertilization. In contrast, ulipristal is supposed to be able to block them at the last minute.

Situation 3: Embryo is Already on its Way to the Uterus

If, however, the sexual contact took place during the ovulation period but the emergency pill is only taken one or two days later, there is a 30% probability that fertilization could have taken place. What possibly happens to the embryo now differs a lot depending on which pill is taken.

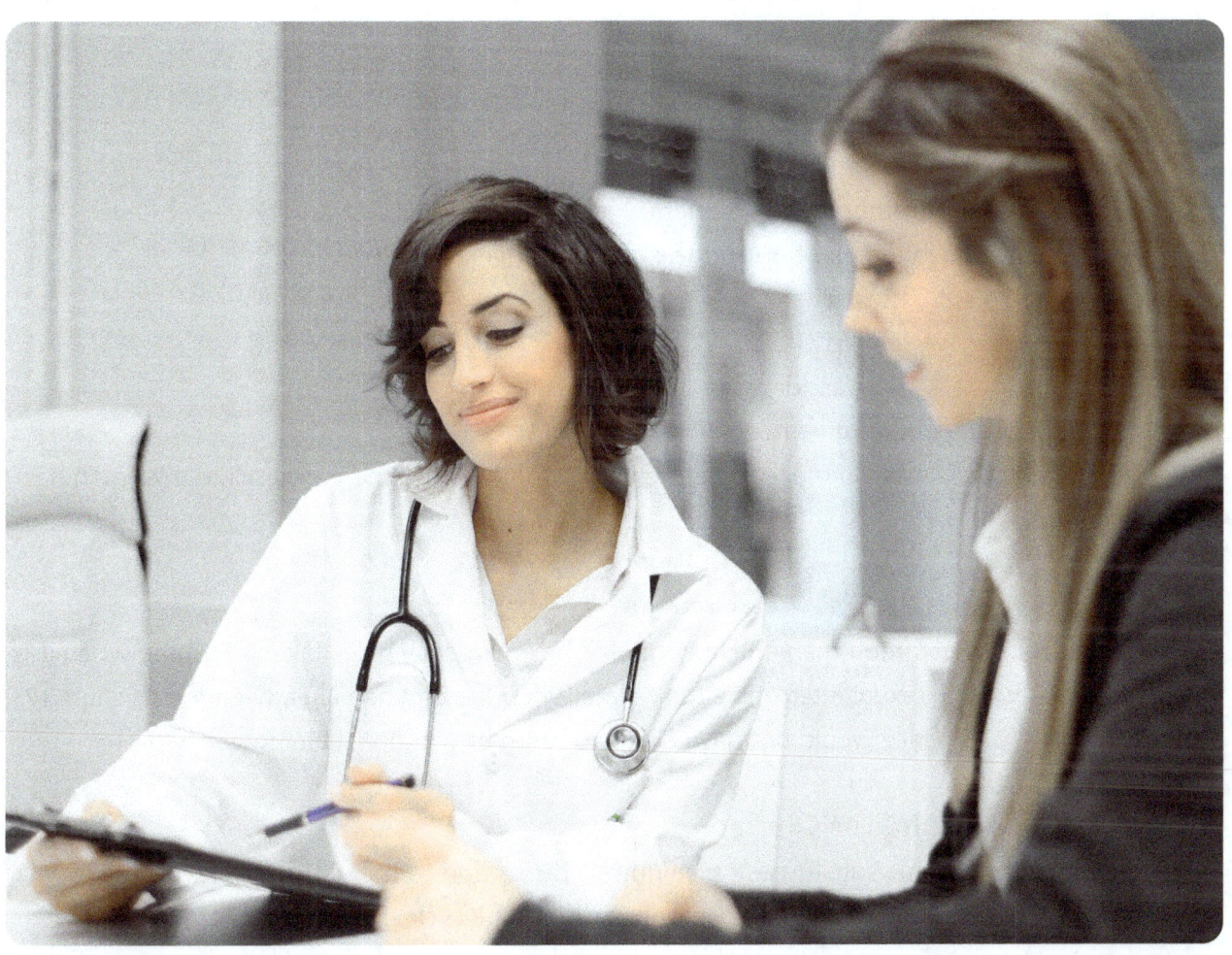

A regular medical check-up is essential in regard to all hormonal contraceptive methods.

Taking Levonorgestrel
Medical studies indicate the chance of survival for the embryo is quite high if levonorgestrel is taken only the second or third day after fertilization. It is already on its way to the uterus, where the corpus luteum has prepared the Luxury Suites for its arrival. If an extra amount of progestogen from the emergency pill reaches the body in this phase, then there appears to be little harm to the embryo. The high number of pregnancies which occur when levonorgestrel has been taken after ovulation indicates the low efficacy when fertilization has already occurred.

Taking Ulipristal Acetate
It is a different situation with ulipristal acetate, which can be taken up to five days after unprotected sexual intercourse. With a 30% chance of fertilization, as mentioned above, an embryo could be traveling to the uterus. If ulipristal acetate is taken at this time, it acts as a progesterone antagonist. The natural progesterone, which was preparing the uterine lining, will be displaced by the "anti-hormone." It takes no responsibility for further preparation, the decoration of the uterine lining is stopped, and the embryo can't implant. The uterine lining is no longer built up and the embryo cannot implant. The mechanism of action of nidation inhibition is very likely here.

> **FACT**
> *It should be noted for both types of emergency pill; the sooner they are taken after unprotected sexual intercourse the more likely it is that it will delay ovulation.*

If ulipristal acetate is taken accidentally during pregnancy, a miscarriage cannot be ruled out. This is why a pregnancy test is recommended before taking this kind of emergency pill, if a woman has missed a period.

Situation 4: Ovulation is Over – Egg No Longer Available
This situation is more common than one may think. The emergency pill is taken at a time when it is totally unnecessary. The sexual intercourse took place when the egg had already ended its short 12 to 18 hour life. A pregnancy would not have occurred, with or without the emergency pill!

Not Suitable as a Method of Contraception
The high doses of hormone substitutes cause quite a disruption to the natural cycle, particularly before ovulation. Sometimes it leads to postponement of the cycle, menstrual disorders, and delayed maturation of the next follicle. This is one of the main reasons it is advised not to use the emergency pill regularly.

11 It's All a Matter of Timing

Those who understand what's going on in a female's cycle know there are only a few days in which a pregnancy can occur. These "fertile days" consist of the few days before ovulation, when the cervical mucus is available and allows the sperm access to the Stage of Life, and the short life of the egg after ovulation.

We speak of the beginning of the cycle, when no cervical mucus is available yet and no eggs are ready to be fertilized, as being the *"infertile phase."*

The second phase of the cycle, following ovulation, is known as the *"completely infertile phase."* There are two reasons for this:

- The Shutdown Agreement prevents further eggs from maturing, so no ovulation can occur.
- The Progesterone Team close the cervix and the cervical mucus dries up, therefore the sperm remain outside.

This knowledge about the fertile and infertile phases in the cycle can be used by a woman or a couple to avoid pregnancy, but also to find out the best possible time to become pregnant. Pretty ingenious really! So why is this knowledge about timing not used more often? The answer is quite simple: It is ingenious, but it is also quite demanding.

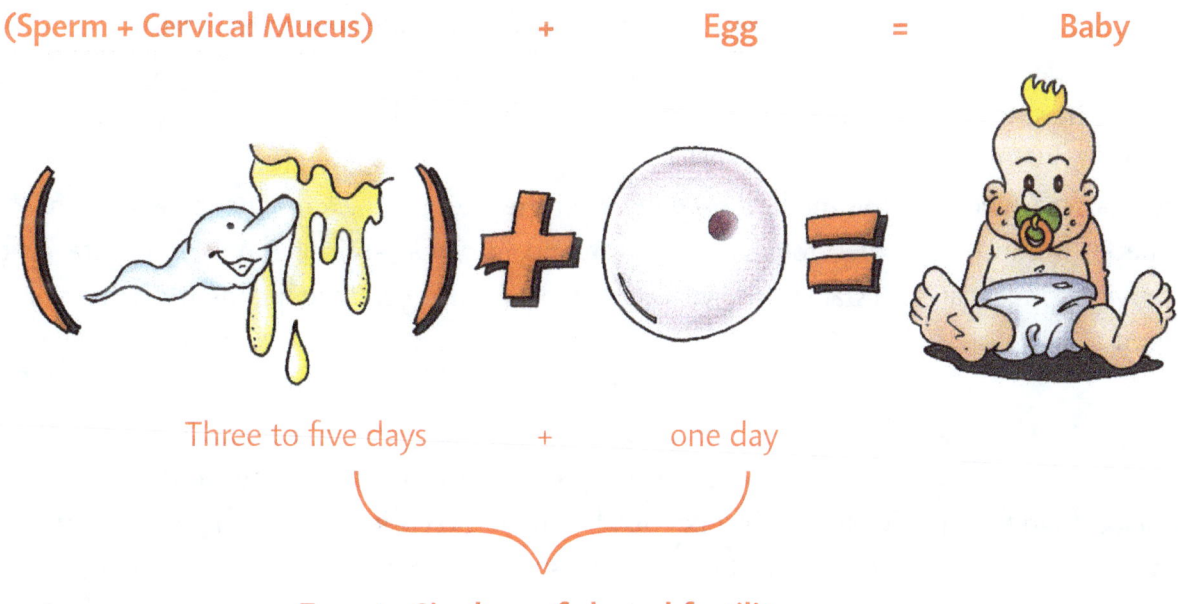

(Sperm + Cervical Mucus)   +   Egg   =   Baby

Three to five days   +   one day

Four to Six days of shared fertility between a man and a woman in one cycle.

Learning Body Language First: If You Know your Body Well, You Can Trust it.

Using "the right timing" to avoid a pregnancy is quite a challenge, because the ability to decipher the body's secret language must first be learned before one can really depend on the timing. More and more women today are well informed and know all about both their menstrual cycle and their own body; some of them are even trained "body language teachers" (natural family planning teachers) who pass on their knowledge and experience to others. Other women exchange views with others on the internet. Perhaps in a few years time it will become quite normal for women to master their body language and to recognize when they are fertile.

Girls and women who find it easiest to learn their body language are those who are able to approach the whole subject calmly because their primary goal is not to avoid a pregnancy. They are curious and want to learn more about themselves; they don't want others telling them what's going on in their own bodies.

Every Method Has its Rules

Anyone hoping to be able to rely on the correct timing to avoid pregnancy must first carefully learn the rules applying to the fertile and infertile days in the menstrual cycle. This method is called "Natural Family Planning" (NFP Method) and refers to a sympto-thermal method, which, if learned correctly, is as effective as the birth control pill.

With the aid of the two most important body codes, the cervical mucus ("sympto") and body temperature ("thermal"), the beginning and end of the fertile phase can be determined.
You can compare learning the right timing with learning to drive. The first step is a learning phase where you have to learn the rules and practice; once learned, you have the knowledge and ability for the rest of your fertile life.

You can teach yourself this method from books or the internet (see end of chapter), but it is even better to consult an expert for advice. You can find your nearest teacher on the websites who will provide support and assistance until you are capable of safely and independently determining the right timing.

"Sex isn't Just the One Thing"

Getting the timing right is demanding, as, naturally, no unprotected sexual intercourse is allowed to take place during the fertile phase, which, depending on the cycle length, is roughly 30 to 50% of the cycle. This means there are times when cool heads have to be kept, despite burning desire.

If two people are depending on the right timing, they can't risk having a mental blackout, even if the situation gets heated between them. They have to make a joint decision of whether or not it is okay to have sexual intercourse. This means talking to each other and consciously taking responsibility for the shared fertility and the Equation of Life. It's about one's own body and the body of the other person; it's about health, love and respect.

When a couple can only think of "just one thing" when they hear the words "love" and "sex", or when there is silence between them when "nothing's going on," then it would probably be completely unsuitable for them to use the right timing method. This method suits imaginative and creative couples much better as they know:

> **FACT**
> There are many ways people try to avoid a pregnancy in a "natural" way. Recently a large number of fertility tracking apps appeared on the market. They could be of some help when a couple wants to have a baby; however, for birth control, most of them are unreliable as they only calculate the fertile phase.

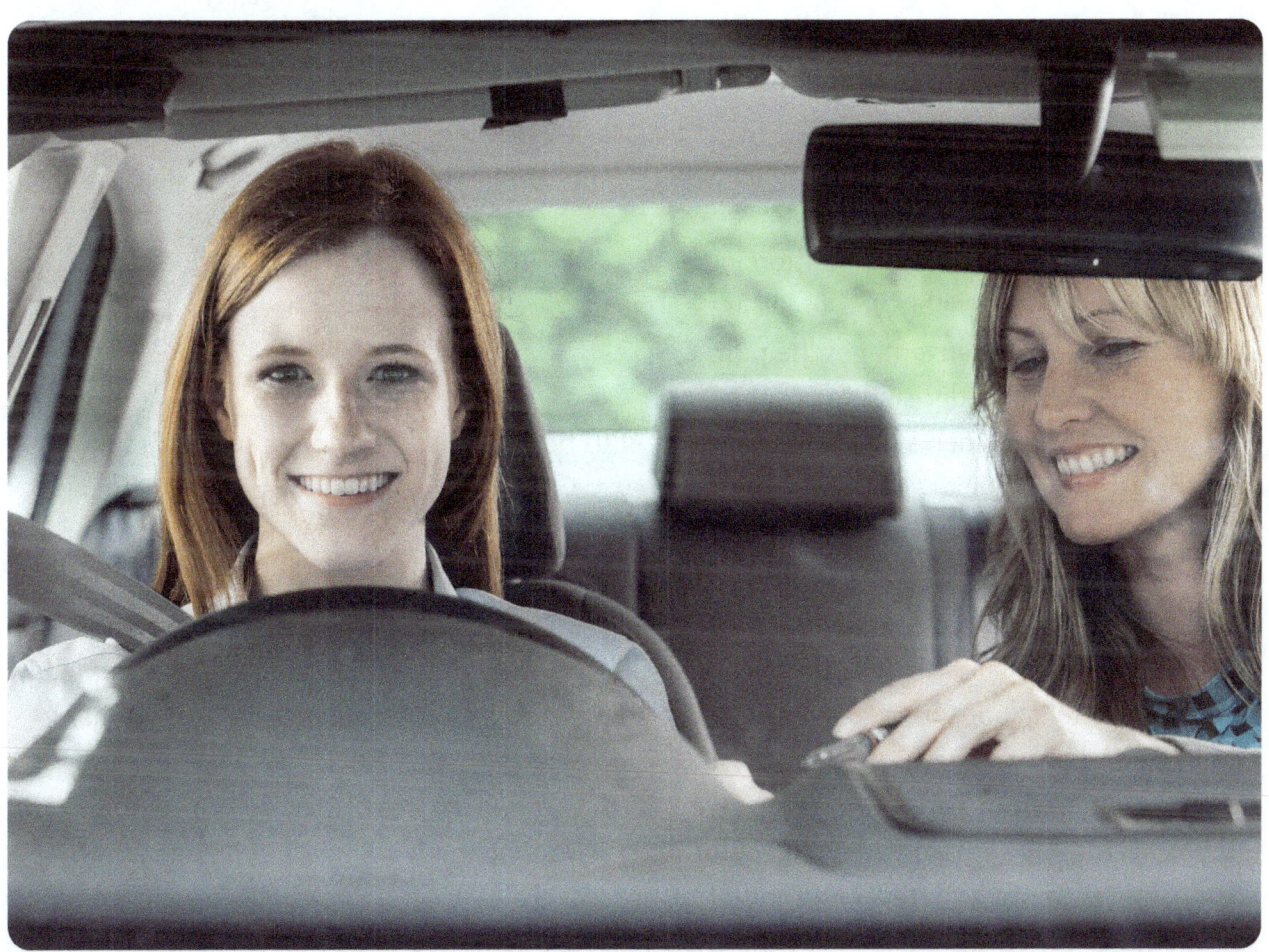

Learning the right timing is similar to learning to drive; once you have the knowledge, you have it for the rest of your life.

- It doesn't mean nothing is happening when "nothing's going on."
- Love is not just sex, and sex is not just sexual intercourse.
- Displaying affection and caressing each other is the most beautiful language of love, and there are many other ways of saying "I love you" with one's body.
- Variety is the spice of life and keeps love alive!
- Highlights only remain highlights when they are not common.

Perhaps Not at the Moment, Maybe Later! There is a Natural and Safe Alternative

It's quite possible that you are not at all enthusiastic about the idea of "becoming slowly acquainted with your body" in your current life situation. Maybe you already have a boyfriend, and like a lot of girls around you, you wish to opt for hormonal contraception. According to widespread public opinion, this is the best method to protect you from an unplanned pregnancy. The information in the previous chapter will enable you to evaluate its advantages and disadvantages, helping you to make the right decision for yourself.

> **FACT**
> *The latest scientific research confirms that the efficacy of the sympto-thermal method ("Sensiplan"), when properly learned and applied, is equal to that of the birth control pill.*

Lots of young women start their fertile life with hormonal contraceptive methods and take them for many years. Many report that they have been more or less happy with their choice, but there was no reliable information about better alternatives. When they encounter the possibility of self-observation of their own body (i.e. the NFP method) years later, they often regret not having discovered it earlier. They are happy now, however, having still had the chance to get familiar with their body, their cycle, and their fertility. They often feel completely different and talk about "understanding themselves much better", enjoying being a woman, and living in harmony with their bodies.

In dealing with the subject of fertility and birth control, choices or decisions once made are not necessarily set for life. New decisions can always be made depending on age and circumstances in life. Whatever method of birth control a woman chooses at a certain time, she should always bear in mind that there is a reliable alternative to avoid pregnancy, which protects a woman's health and her precious fertility.

Information on the MFM Project

A Pioneering Fertility Awareness Project to Accompany Girls, Boys and Their Parents Through Puberty.

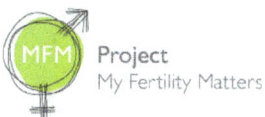

How girls experience and value their own bodies has a huge influence on their self image and self esteem. It is one of the most decisive developmental tasks to accept oneself and experience the physical changes of puberty in a positive way. The better young girls are prepared for this challenge, the better they can later deal with their fertility and sexuality.

"I Can Only Protect What I Value and Respect."

This was the guiding principle for Elisabeth Raith-Paula, MD when she set up the MFM Project in Germany in 1999. When taught about their fertility many of her adult female patients had asked "Why haven't we been told this before?" which gave Elisabeth Raith-Paula, MD the insight to write a book to teach young girls about the signs of fertility. Parent evenings were later set up to help them understand their daughter's pending puberty, and during these sessions it was suggested that there should be a one day training program to teach the girls. From this request emerged this large, popular European project; which also includes the boys' workshop.

Since 1999, the demand for the MFM Project has grown rapidly, reaching more than half a billion girls, boys, and parents. In 2002, the MFM Project was awarded the prestigious Bavarian health promotion and disease prevention award; in 2003, it was awarded a "best practice project" of the European Union; and in 2004, it received a scholarship in counseling (Start-Social McKinsey). In November 2012, Dr. Raith-Paula became an Ashoka Fellow. (www.ashoka.org)

Currently, in Germany, more than 330 active trainers are running workshops, mainly in schools. In 2017, over 70,000 girls, boys, and their parents were reached by more than 5000 project events in Germany.

Meanwhile, the MFM project has spread to many countries (France, Austria, Switzerland, England, Hungary, Belgium, Latvia, Lithuania, Mauritius, Ivory Coast, China, Australia, Mexico and the United States.)

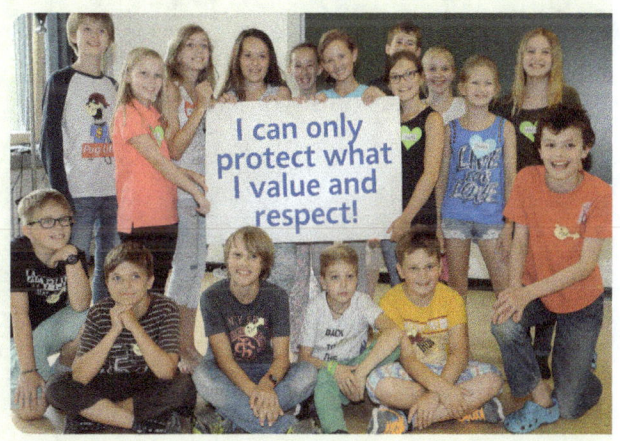

Information on the Guiding Star Cycle Show Workshop

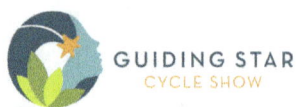

A Workshop for Girls aged 9-12 Years

The Cycle Show is an educational, interactive, multi-media, fertility awareness workshop for young girls. It is a desirable addition to the standard sex education given in schools; its aim is to equip young girls with the knowledge of what is going on inside their bodies in relation to puberty. This knowledge then supports and prepares them in a positive way for the wonderful changes they will experience within their bodies over the coming years.

Today it is more important than ever for young girls to have high self esteem regarding their bodies, not just when they are in the middle of puberty, but before the onset. The beginning of sexual maturation is the ideal time for girls to learn about and appreciate all the amazing changes that are taking place within their bodies. Participation in the Cycle Show gives girls a healthy respect for their bodies and helps to protect them as they move into their teenage years.

Language and Images Used

All language and images used within the workshop must come from the trademarked script supplied by the International MFM Project. The script is followed by all trainers to ensure that biological terms are always used simultaneously with positive images or comparisons and is respectful of the age and innocence of the girls attending the Cycle Show.

What Happens During a Cycle Show Workshop?

The Cycle Show illustrates to girls what is happening inside a woman's body in a loving and respectful way, using colorful materials, scarves, music, and fun games.

In the first part of the work-shop the girls are introduced to the "Equation of Life" (Sperm + Egg = New Life). The girls themselves take on the roles

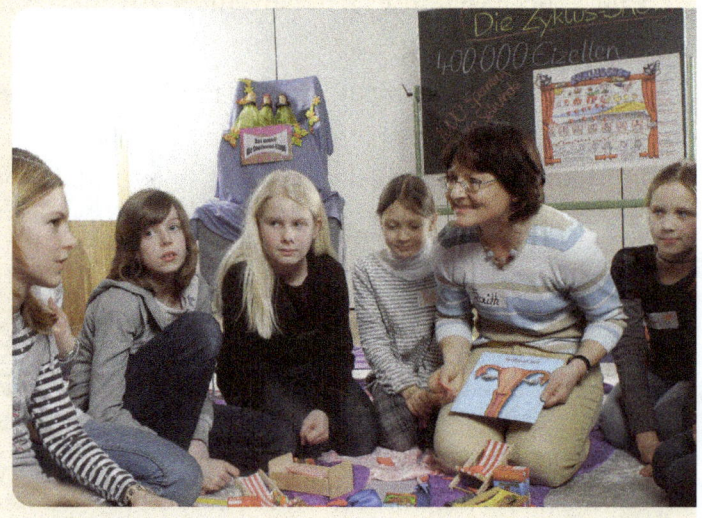

of hormones and experience how the Messengers of Spring (FSH), the Estrogen Friends, the Ovulation Helpers (LH), and Progesterone Team work in the body of a woman to create human life.

After gaining a basic knowledge of the actions of the hormones and seeing them as her friends, the second and main part of the workshop is focused on each girl understanding how these hormones act within her own body. She learns that with each cycle, a new Luxury Suite (lining of the uterus) is prepared for a potential guest (baby), and if the guest doesn't arrive (and shouldn't for her until she is older), she will not worry about the loss of the Luxury Suite, knowing that each month her body prepares a new one because her healthy body can afford it.

Finally, the girls recognize fertility codes within their bodies, such as the Magic Potion (cervical mucus). Menstrual hygiene options are discussed, and girls are taught what to expect and how to manage their first bleed.

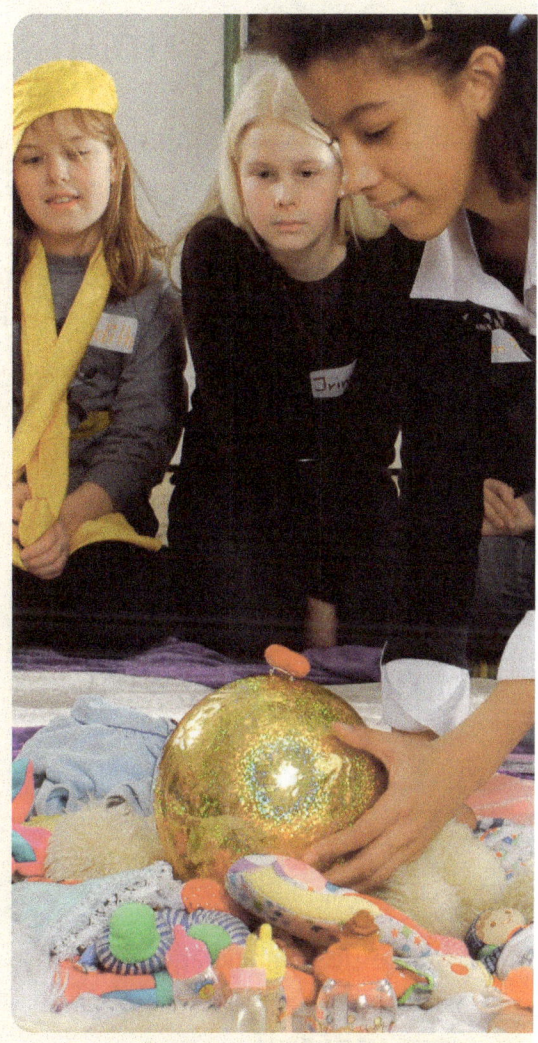

Why Choose a Guiding Star Cycle Show?

Like a theatre audience staring at the red curtains that frame an empty dark stage, waiting for something to happen, many women in our society do the same for their menstrual period. They are completely unaware of what actually takes place in their bodies leading up to menstruation. We explain these events in an impressive behind the scenes show.

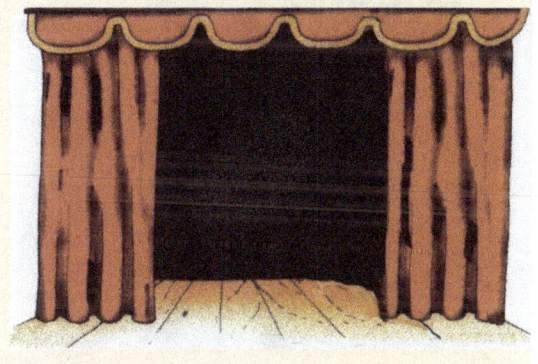

Further Information

For further information regarding the Guiding Star Cycle Show, how to register, or to learn how become a trained instructor, please scan the code below or email the Guiding Star Cycle Show National Coordinator directly at **cycleshow@theguidingstarproject.com**. Cycle Show is also an international program and known in many countries. To learn more about the project visit: **www.mfm-projekt.eu**

The Boys Project – Agents on a Mission

A Fertility Workshop for Boys recommended for ages 10-11 years

The similar project for boys has been running since 2003. In the workshop "Agents on a Mission," the boys discover what's going on in their bodies during puberty. They explore how new life comes into existence as well as what's happening in the girls bodies, all in a fun, respectful, and age appropriate manner.

To learn more about the history of how the Cycle Show came to be and the development of The Boys Project–Agents on a Mission watch this video on YouTube: "Royal College Video"

Important Terms and Definitions

Amenorrhoea: Absence of a menstrual period in a woman of reproductive age for more than 90 days.

Androgens: Collective term for male sexual hormones.

Anorexia nervosa: An eating disorder characterized by low weight, fear of gaining weight, and food restriction. It is always associated with amenorrhea.

Cervical mucus: Secretion from the cervical glands, and stimulated by the estrogen some days prior to and around ovulation. It is the most important fertility sign and essential for sperm nutrition and survival.

Cervix: Lower part of the uterus (2-3cm/about 1in.) containing glands for the production of the cervical mucus. Here sperm can survive up to 5 days.

Chromosome: DNA molecule containing the genetic material. Humans have 46 chromosomes.

COC/ Birth Control Pill: The combined oral contraceptive pill is a birth control method that includes a combination of synthetic substitutes of estrogen and progesterone (= progestin).

Corpus luteum: This gland develops from the ovarian follicle after ovulation and produces progesterone.

Corpus luteum deficiency: Limited function of the corpus luteum.

Discharge (vaginal discharge): Most discharge represents normal functioning of the body (especially estrogen induced cervical mucus). Some can reflect infection or other pathological processes typically associated with bad odor, itching, or pain.

Ejaculation (seminal discharge): The discharge of seminal fluid from the penis.

Embryo: The earliest stage in the development of a fertilized egg (the zygote) i.e. human life in the first three months after fertilization.

Epididymis: A paired organ in the male reproductive system where sperm are stored and undergo a 2-3 month maturation process.

Estrogen: Group of three female sex hormones which are produced mainly in the ovarian follicle and which have numerous effects within the woman`s body. At puberty, they are jointly responsible for the development of the female physical features.

Fallopian tubes: A pair of very fine tubes measuring around 4-6 in., connecting the top of the uterus on both sides to the ovaries. The finger-shaped fringe ends place themselves over the follicle before ovulation and catch the egg. Fertilization takes place near the fimbriated end of the fallopian tube. The fertilized egg travels towards the uterus aided by activity of the tubal cilia and tubal muscle.

Fertilization: Fusion of sperm and egg to initiate the development of a new human being.

Fimbriae: Finger-shaped fringes of the fallopian tubes,

Important Terms and Definitions

which place themselves over the ovary to catch the egg during ovulation.

Follicle: Protective cover around the egg in the ovary. It secretes estrogens during the first part of the menstrual cycle.

Follicle stimulating hormone (FSH): Hormone which is produced and secreted by the pituitary gland. It triggers the egg ripening.

Follicular phase: First phase of the menstrual cycle in which the egg matures in the ovary. It ends with ovulation.

Glands: Organs that generate hormones or other substances and release them into the blood or other body canals.

Hormones: Hormones are often produced by glands and are our body's chemical messengers. They travel in the bloodstream to tissues or organs and affect many different processes.

Human chorionic gonadotropin (hCG): Hormone produced by the placenta after implantation of the embryo. It enters the mother's bloodstream and can be detected in a pregnancy test.

Hymen: Membrane that surrounds or partially covers the external vaginal opening.

Hypothalamus: It is located in the brain and among other things is responsible for the secretion of "releasing hormones" which stimulate or inhibit the secretion of pituitary hormones.

Implantation: The process of the embryo becoming attached to the prepared uterine lining, roughly about a week after fertilization.

Intermenstrual bleeding: Bleeding from the vagina which has nothing to do with the normal period. It takes place "out of order" and can have diverse, sometimes pathological reasons.

Luteal phase: Second phase of the menstrual cycle following ovulation in which the corpus luteum hormone, progesterone, is preparing the woman's body for a possible pregnancy.

Luteinizing hormone (LH): Hormone from the pituitary gland. The acute rise triggers ovulation and the development of the corpus luteum.

Menarche: A girl's first menstrual period

Menstruation (period): A regularly recurring bleeding from the vagina in women of child-bearing age, caused by the bleeding of the upper layer of the uterine lining.

Mini pill: Another name for the progestogen only pill (POP) with no synthetic estrogen substitute.

Monophasic cycle: Cycle with no progesterone induced rise in temperature; ovulation does not usually occur.

Important Terms and Definitions

Natural family planning (NFP): Natural birth control method. The fertile and infertile phase is determined by observing the body's signs, especially cervical mucus changes and body temperature. For safe use, certain rules have to be learned and adhered to.

Ovaries: The two female sexual glands, found in the pelvis. From puberty to menopause, the eggs mature here and the female sex hormones estrogen and progesterone are produced.

Ovulation: It is the release of the egg from the ovary.

Ovulation bleeding: Rare, usually slight bleeding (intermenstrual bleeding), which occurs around ovulation, probably associated with the decline of estrogen concentration around ovulation.

Ovulation pain: Abdominal pain which occurs around ovulation. It is associated with the high concentration of estrogen at that time.

Pituitary gland: This endocrine gland is located at the base of the brain and regulates several physiological processes and the function of many other hormonal glands in the body.

Pregnancy test: Blood or urine test to detect a pregnancy as early as 10 to 16 days after fertilization, when the embryo has attached to the uterine lining. Then human chorionic gonadotropin (hCG) is present in the mother's blood and urine.

Premenstrual syndrome (PMS): Physical and mental changes of varying intensity which occur in the second phase of the menstrual cycle, often a few days before the next period and disappear when the period starts. The cause is still largely not understood.

Progesterone: Female sex hormone which is produced in the corpus luteum in the ovary after ovulation. It prepares the woman's body for a pregnancy. If conception has occurred, the progesterone maintains the pregnancy.

Progestogen: Collective term for a number of synthetic substitutes for the natural progesterone (also called progestins).

Proliferation phase: First cycle phase in which, stimulated by the estrogen, the upper layer of the uterine lining is rebuilt again.

Prostate: It is the largest gland of the male sex organs and lies beneath the bladder. It acts like a gate that stops the sperm and the urine from mixing. It releases a slightly alkaline fluid into the vas during ejaculation. This secretion makes up the main part of the seminal fluid and supports sperm mobility.

Puberty: Phase of development between childhood and adulthood, accompanied by physical and emotional changes.

Secretion phase: Second phase of the menstrual cycle when, after ovulation, progesterone from the corpus luteum prepares the uterine lining for a possible implantation of an embryo.

Seminal vesicles: Both vesicle glands flow into the vas, providing the sperm with a nutritious fluid containing fructose and vitamin C.

Sex hormones: Collective term for the hormones that are formed in the woman's ovaries (estrogen and progesterone) and in the man's testicles (androgens).

Sperm: Male germ cell (gamete), sperm cell, spermatozoa.

Spotting: Slight bleeding from the vagina occurs whereby underwear can be stained reddish brown. Some women experience spotting shortly before the start of their period, it occurs more frequently when using the copper coil or hormonal contraceptive methods.

Sympto-thermal Method: Natural method of birth control in which the woman observes her body codes and chooses "the right timing," i.e. determines the fertile time, by changes in temperature and cervical mucus.

Testicles (Testis): These are the male gonads which produce the sperm and the male sex hormone, testosterone.

Testosterone: The primary male sex hormone mainly produced in the testicles.

Withdrawal: Very unreliable contraceptive method, also known as "coitus interruptus," in which a man withdraws his penis from the woman's vagina prior to ejaculation.I

Index

A

amenorrhoea 106 ff., 123

androgen 120

B

breast symptom 87, 88

C

cervical gland 20, 24, 37. 50, 73 ff., 113, 124

cervical mucus 23 ff., 36 f., 39, 48, 50 f., 73-77, 95, 99, 104

cervix 20, 36. 39, 82 ff.

chemical messenger 29

clitoris 82

chromosomes 13, 26

condom 109

contraceptive implant 124 f.

contraceptive methods 109 -130

copper intrauterine device 126 f.

corpus luteum 38, 41 ff., 52, 87

D

desogestrel containing POP 122

diaphragm 110

E

egg 15 ff., 19, 25 f., 28 f., 31 f., 34 f.

ejaculation 14, 20, 83

emergency pill 128-130

enzyme 13

estrogen 18, 34-37. 47-52, 64 f., 74, 76, 84 ff., 103 f., 107, 111, 116-118, 125

F

fallopian tube 17, 19, 25, 28, 31, 37. 85, 127

fertilization 26 ff.

fertility 9 ff., 32, 91-99, 119, 134
follicle 34 ff.
follicular phase 38, 94 f., 107
FSH (follicular stimulating hormone) 34, 44, 47, 107

H
hymen 20, 69, 82
hypothalamus 33, 46, 111

I
implantation 29, 127
intermenstrual bleeding 86 f., 113, 115, 125
intra uterine system 122

L
LH (luteinizing hormone) 36 f., 104
luteal phase 40, 105 ff.,

M
mammary glands 40, 87
menarche 52-57
menstruation 34 f., 48, 58 ff.
messenger substance 18, 64
mini pill 122

N
natural family planning 132-135
negative feedback mechanism 41, 111, 121, 123 f.

O
ovarian inflammation 86
ovary 15, 16 ff., 35, 111
ovulation 16, 25, 31, 35 ff., 41, 44, 76, 80 ff., 103, 107, 116
ovulation bleeding 86
ovulation pain 85 f.

P
panty liners 61, 70
period 19, 31, 35, 40, 52-70
pituitary gland 33, 37. 111
premenstrual syndrome (PMS) 90
progesterone 18, 38 ff., 41, 43 ff., 52, 65, 78-82, 87 f., 104 f., 112, 117
progestogen 111, 112, 120 ff., 128
progestogen only injection 121, 123

S
sanitary pad 64, 68 ff.
seminal vesicle 14
spotting 123, 125
sympto-thermal method 132, 134

T
tampons 68 ff., 73
testicles 12-14
testosterone 120
tubal pregnancy 127
twenty-eight day cycle 91-96, 119

U
uterine lining 35, 43, 112 ff.
uterus 18 ff., 21-25, 28-31, 50 f.

V
vagina 17, 20-22, 68, 73 ff., 83
von Willebrand disease 53

W
withdrawal 110
withdrawal bleeding 114

Additional Resources

- **FertilityCare**: List of teachers of the Creighton Model system, as well as doctors who practice NaProTechnology® around the country —https://fertilitycare.org/find-a-mc

- **FACTS About Fertility**: Group of physicians, healthcare professionals and educators working together to provide information about natural or fertility awareness based methods of family planning with the medical community. — https://www.factsaboutfertility.org/

- **FEMM:** Comprehensive women's health and wellness program for optimal reproductive health. Offers a natural, breakthrough, science-based program to help women learn more about their bodies, and how to identify daily hormonal shifts to achieve their health and fertility goals. https://femmhealth.org

- **SymptoPro:** Sympto-Thermal Method of fertility charting, based on changes in a woman's cervical mucus, waking or resting temperature, and cervix—https://guidingstarproject.com/online-fertility-education-with-symptopro/

- **Billings Method:** Fertility awareness-based method (FABM) of family planning that relies on the observation of patterns of fertility and infertility based on vulvar sensations and appearance of discharges—https://boma-usa.org

- **Marquette Method:** Form of Natural Family Planning (NFP) that uses Clearblue Fertility Monitors to track women's urinary biomarkers—estrogen and luteinizing hormone levels—to precisely identify the fertile window in each menstrual cycle.—https://vitaefertility.com

- **Creighton Method:** Fertility awareness method that relies upon the standardized observation and charting of biological markers that are essential to a woman's health and fertility. —https://creightonmodel.com

- **Managing Your Fertility:** Fertility awareness resources—https://managingyourfertility.com

- **The Saint Paul VI Institute:** Provides support for infertility, NaProTechnology®, and women's health—https://popepaulvi.com

- **The Fertility Awareness Database:** Resources for fertility awareness based methods and links to instructors across the country—https://fabmbase.org

- **Whole Mission:** Resources for the Marquette Method of fertility charting and directory of charting instructors—https://www.mmnfp.com/

- **The Guiding Star Project:** We help women protect their fertility and identity as mothers through our sisterhood of life-affirming birth centers—lighting the way to a culture of life. —https://guidingstarproject.com.

- **Pro Women's Healthcare Centers**: Affiliated centers provide comprehensive, convenient, compassionate, high-quality medical services and access to social services that empower women to care for their health—https://pwhc.org

- **Natural Womanhood:** Promotes fertility awareness and natural family planning as essential tools for women's health, and as natural birth control alternatives.— https://naturalwomanhood.org/

- **Happy Girl's Guide to Being Whole, What you Never Knew Abour Your Natural Body:** Written by, Teresa Kenney, WHP, she walks you through the basic knowledge of your female body—everything you never knew. Recommended for ages 16-24 as a way to further educate yourself on your changing female body.—https://www.lumenpress.org/

www.ingramcontent.com/pod-product-compliance
Lightning Source LLC
Chambersburg PA
CBHW080838230426
43665CB00021B/2880